MW01235349

# Answering the Call

*Inspirational Devotionals from a Tested Paramedic*

A Christian Devotions Ministries publication

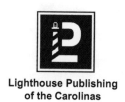

**Lighthouse Publishing
of the Carolinas**

# Answering the Call

Published by Christian Devotions Ministry,
P. O. Box 6494, Kingsport, TN, 37663
ChristianDevotions.us • answeringthecall.us

Our mission is to publish inspirational products that touch the heart,
minister to the soul, and glorify God. All scripture quotations,
unless otherwise indicated, are taken from the
HOLY BIBLE, NEW INTERNATIONAL VERSION®. NIV®.
Copyright © 1973, 1978, 1984 by International Bible Society.
Used by permission of Zondervan. All rights reserved.
Published in association with Lighthouse Publishing of the Carolinas.

Available direct from your local bookstore, online,
or from the publisher at: christiandevotionsbooks.com

Book Cover and Interior Design by Behind the Gift.
• behindthegift.com

ISBN-13: 978-0-9822065-3-9  ISBN-10: 0-9822065-3-4

Printed in the United States of America.

# Dedication

This book is dedicated to my old friend
## Andrew James Stocks
Marine, Firefighter, Paramedic, Teacher, Soldier, and finally
N.C. State Trooper.

You died in the line of duty on September 9, 2008.
Gave your life that another might live. You are no longer
with us but your memory lives on. God bless you,
my friend. I know where you are and I'll see you again.
Until then, "Medic-7 is supersonic. We'll be there in
30-seconds!"

# Forward

First Responders are always waiting. Ready and willing to sacrifice their own comfort and safety in order to protect others. I know. I was one. As a street medic I served with firefighters and police officers, emergency medical technicians and other paramedics, dedicated men and women who were willing to give their all. And together we made a profound difference. We touched, helped, counseled and saved more people than I can recall. We witnessed violence and grief. Felt victory and defeat. We saw people at their worst, rarely at their best. We laughed with many, cried with a few, saw some born, and watched others die. Over the years we carried home more pain than our minds could reasonably absorb, and many of us had to force ourselves to carry on despite the mental scars that threatened to break us down.

So after twenty years of service—of racing to calls, of plugging bleeding wounds, of starting IV's and pushing drugs, of dealing with death, and witnessing new life—I have come to the following conclusion: The most important aspect of my job was the people. My patients. My partners. My fellow First Responders. Everyone needs love. We long for the human touch. And sometimes all we really need is for another person to listen to us, or to say, "It's okay," and point us in the right direction.

# Answering the Call

Within the pages of Answering the Call, you'll find true stories. Real situations and encounters from my days with EMS. Most are from the street, others from my personal life, but each reflects a profound moment when I heard God's voice echoing quietly in my ear.

As you read each devotional try to place yourself within the context of the story. Consider the underlying problem and the resolution at the end. Then pray for God's guidance as you work through the short series of questions that follow. Open your Bible and read the verses provided. Find out what God has to say to you. I have given you plenty of room for personal notes and prayers.

Finally, if you don't know Jesus Christ I encourage you to drop to your knees today. Confess your failures to him and ask him to become your Savior and Lord. If you already know him, I encourage you to follow him more closely. Either way, I pray that God will perform a mighty work in your life, meet you where you are, and draw ever closer to your side. And that you will respond to His voice, for sooner or later we all must decide for ourselves. There is no hiding from the truth—Jesus Christ is Lord.

"Choose for yourselves this day whom you will serve—but as for me and my household, we will serve the LORD."
Joshua 24:15

# Respond!
# Your life depends on it!

Here I am! I stand at the door and knock. If anyone hears my voice and opens the door, I will come
in and eat with him, and he with me.
Revelation 3:20

Imagine if you called for help and nobody responded.
How terrified would it make you feel to realize you
were all alone? Well what I'm speaking of here is eternity.
Jesus wants to come into your life. Have you heard Him
knocking? Have you responded yet? Opened the door?

"C'mon, partner, we need to go!"

"Unh uh, I'm not going."

"Right," I said with a chuckle. "Put your boots on, man. I'll
be in the truck."

"I'm serious. I wanna see the end of this game."

I gazed at my partner trying to see the humor in what
appeared to be a sick joke. "You what?"

# Answering the Call

"Medic-seven?" the dispatcher exclaimed. The station radio crackled as if to emphasize the frustration in her voice. "Are you en route yet?"

"Don't answer it," my partner said leaning forward to watch a long fly ball.

"We can't just ignore it," I said. "We have to go!"

"Look, I'm not wasting my time on another silly call. It's a cardiac arrest for crying out loud. There's probably nothing we can do for the poor guy anyway."

The radio crackled again. "Medic-seven?"

"Medic-seven to dispatch," I said. "Stand by please." I turned to my partner. "Are you insane? Do you realize what you're doing?"

"Sure I do."

*"Medic-seven!"*

"Seven," I said keying my lapel mike. "I-I'm sorry, but you'll have to send another unit. It's my partner, he's…he's refusing to take this call."

A few seconds of uncomfortable silence passed before the radio erupted in a swarm of heated responses— the dispatcher, our supervisor, the fire department first responders already en route to the scene—everyone fighting for radio space, trying to make some sense of what they'd just heard. I glanced at my partner. He sat in front the television casually watching the game.

"I can't believe you're gonna just sit there. Someone's life is on the line."

*"Relax," he said. "Sit down and watch the game. If we ignore it, it'll all just go away."*

Sound ridiculous? Well don't worry, it'll never happen. First Responders are some of the most dedicated people I know. They jump into action whenever the tones sound, regardless of the weather or time of day. They do it for others, and as a result lives are saved. And yet I wonder, do these people care as much for themselves as they do for their patients? Do you?

Jesus said, "Here I am! I stand at the door and knock." He wants to come into your life. To bring you salvation, peace, and joy. Don't ignore him. Respond without delay. Because someone's life is on the line. Yours!

# PRAYER

Thank you for First Responders everywhere, those men and women who risk their own lives every day that others might live. I pray for their safety, for their judgment, for their salvation. They need to care for themselves, Lord. Give them the courage to open that door.

## APPLICATION

Have you ever found yourself in that situation? Where you cried for help and no one responded? Well when it comes to eternity you have nothing to fear, for Jesus Christ is knocking at your door. Read the scripture heading again. What does he promise to do if you will open the door?

Now open your Bible and read John 14:23. What else does Christ promise to those who love him and obey his commands?

And John 3:16. What gift does Christ promise to whomsoever would believe in him?

Have you made the decision to open the door and allow the Lord Jesus Christ into your life? If not will you do so today?

## BUILDING BLOCKS OF FAITH

Jesus Christ is knocking—Open the door to your heart and let Him in.

# Answering the Call

## JOURNAL

_____

_____

_____

_____

_____

_____

_____

_____

_____

_____

_____

_____

_____

_____

_____

_____

_____

_____

# A Good Drunk

*"If you love those who love you, what reward will you get? Are not even the tax collectors doing that?"*
Matthew 5:46

Yeah I'm a Christian, but I had me a good drunk the other night.

No, really. I found him lying in the middle of the street, bump on his head and a bottle of booze by his side. He was about fifty something, dressed in simple clothes and stinking like a sack of dirty laundry. With slurred speech and the sweet, slushy scent of cheap alcohol lingering on his breath, he was about as common as can get. A real good drunk.

I chuckled. I'm a paramedic. I've seen it all before. It should have been a simple call—pick him up, throw him on the stretcher, and give him a ride to the ER for observation, oh, and by the way, pray for him—but it wasn't that easy. He became belligerent. Then he wanted to fight me. Then he went and opened his mouth. I won't tell you what he said. Christians don't use words like that. Or do we?

# Answering the Call

I know I should have held my tongue but before I could think I flung the words right back at him. After all, he deserved it. I was only trying to help him. Right?

Perhaps, but I was wrong. Dead wrong.

You know, I've been a Christian for over thirty years, and you'd think by now I'd know better, but for me it's not that simple. I seem to make one mistake after another, failing the Lord in so many areas of my life that recently a thought has been heavy on my mind:

What does it really mean to be a Christian?

Does it mean never missing church? Attending the right Bible studies? Smiling at other people and never uttering a foul word? I believe Jesus answered my question when He said, "Love your enemies, and pray for those who persecute you." Loving those who **do not** love you is the mark of a true Christian.

"But, Lord?" I ask. "How can I love that guy?"

If I close my eyes, I can picture Jesus hanging on the cross. If I use my imagination, I can see myself kneeling at His bloody feet. But if I put aside my pride, my arrogance, and my selfish ambitions, I can imagine that man kneeling by my side—dirty clothes, stinking breath and all—and suddenly I realize this simple truth: We're both sinners. Christ died for both of us.

# Answering the Call

Now imagine yourself kneeling at the cross. That gnarly piece of upright timber drips red with your savior's blood. And beside you kneels another person…that co-worker or supervisor or arrogant family member you so detest. Look at them. Do you see them? Christ died for that person, just as He died for you. So keep His commandment. Love them. It's what He called you to do.

I failed my test last Saturday night, but Jesus used that failure to teach me a valuable lesson. He showed me what it really means to be a Christian…and He used a good drunk to do it.

## PRAYER

"Lord, I have rejected you and hurled insults at you, and still you love me. Help me to treat others the same way you treat me, with forgiveness, with compassion, and with unconditional Christ-like love."

# Answering the Call

## APPLICATION

Jesus Christ suffered a violent and bloody death so that you might live forever, and all He really asks is that you love others in return. But some people are hard to love, and you can never predict when they will cross your path. But you can be ready for them. Take a few moments now to better prepare yourself. Start by describing a personal encounter with an offensive or unlovable person.

How did that person make you feel?

Did you respond appropriately, or in looking back do you regret your actions?

Read Matthew 5:43-48. What does Christ say about dealing with those who offend you?

Now read 1 Peter 3:9. What is the Christian told not to do?

With these scripture passages in mind, how might you prepare yourself for a similar encounter with that same person or another hard-to-love individual?

# BUILDING BLOCKS OF FAITH

Love your neighbor as yourself.  Do not return evil for
evil.  Christ died that all might live, not just you.

## JOURNAL

_____

_____

_____

_____

_____

_____

_____

_____

_____

_____

_____

_____

_____

_____

_____

_____

# Just Say It, I Dare You!

*"At the name of Jesus every knee should bow and every tongue confess, Jesus Christ is Lord."*
Phil 2:9-11

When I first saw her I thought she was a ghost. She lay beneath a pile of bloody sheets, her wrists opened by a crisscrossed pattern of oozing lashes. With pasty white skin and a fixed unseeing gaze, she looked beyond help, a lost spirit in a living corpse drained of blood. Her name was Noel. She wanted to die. I knelt beside the bed and took her hand. The bones felt limp, the skin cool and dry. A weak pulse throbbed within her wrist. I aligned my face with hers. Her red-rimmed eyes seemed to peer right through me as if I weren't even there. I felt a dark, foreboding presence. Death loomed everywhere.

"Leave me," she whispered. "Can't you see I want to die?"

I dressed her wounds and explained that whether or not she agreed to the transport, I would be taking her to the hospital. The law required it. "And you need to be where people care," I added.

"No one cares."

# Answering the Call

"I care. Look," I said, "come with me. My partner will give us an easy ride."

I saw her hand tremble. She shook her head.

"All we'll do is talk. I promise. Maybe even say a prayer."

She cocked her head and gazed at me. I had hit a nerve.

I wanted to tell her more—that there was someone else who really did care about her, someone who could make a real difference in her life—but I felt a dozen sets of eyes staring at the back of my head. I glanced about the room. Everyone was listening—my fellow rescue workers, the police officers, the girl's family. I suddenly felt like a coward. My tongue wouldn't move. I heard a voice within say, "Be bold, man. Just say it!" But I couldn't say it.

"Come on," I said, standing and snapping my fingers. I felt foolish, angry with myself. "Let's go."

Noel climbed out of bed and padded softly across the room. I positioned her on the stretcher, covered her with a clean sheet, and rolled her to the ambulance praying silently as I walked. *God, give me courage. Please give me courage.*

I kept my word en route to the hospital. No IV bags were spiked. No medications were pushed. All we did was talk. But as we shared I felt a growing need to tell her more. And this time we were alone. My courage grew, but still

# Answering the Call

I felt my pulse begin to race. A hard lump grew in my throat. Why is it so difficult to say that name?

"Noel," I said, my voice low almost in a whisper. "I need to tell you something. Someone does care for you, you know."

"Who?" she exclaimed a pleading expression wrinkling her pale white face. "Please tell me."

"The Lord..." I murmured my heart racing. I could feel myself blushing. My hands began to sweat. "Jesus."

"Huh?" she said lifting a shoulder. "I didn't hear you."

I suddenly realized new strength. I felt my courage grow. I gathered myself and took a deep breath. "Jesus," I said. His name is *Jesus!*"

I saw my partner's jaw drop when he opened the rear doors of the ambulance a few moments later. For Noel looked different. Her previously washed out face appeared bright and pink. Her eyes looked focused and confident.

"What happened," Kevin said, unlocking the stretcher and pulling it from the truck.

# Answering the Call

"I prayed," Noel said taking my hand, "and I know what I need to do now…I need to live. I need to tell other people about Jesus!"

It's been over five years since that night, and I haven't seen Noel since, but I know with certainty that she was transformed in the back of that ambulance, washed clean by the blood of the Lamb. And something else happened too—I was changed forever. For the first time in my life I understood the importance of boldness, of saying His name without fear. There is no other name under Heaven whereby men must be saved.

Do you know Jesus? Do you want to make a difference in someone else's life? Then say it. Be bold and just say it. Like me, you may be surprised by the power unleashed by His name.

## PRAYER

"Heavenly Father, give me the courage to proclaim your Son's wonderful name, to be confident and bold, and to confess to others what I truly believe—Jesus Christ is Lord."

## APPLICATION

The Bible says there is power in the name of Jesus, wonderful life-saving power. Have you ever been frightened to utter his name? Or amazed by the emotion his name seems to evoke? Describe a situation where you were forced to deal with the name, Jesus.

How did you feel at that moment? Did you feel nervous? Angry? Confused?

Read Philippians 2: 5-11. What does this passage have to say about the significance of Christ's name?

What does the Bible say should happen at the mention of his name?

Is there anyone on your heart right now? Someone you know that needs to hear the name, Jesus?

## BUILDING BLOCKS OF FAITH

There is only one name under Heaven whereby men must be saved—Jesus Christ.

# JOURNAL

_____

_____

_____

_____

_____

_____

_____

_____

_____

_____

_____

_____

_____

_____

_____

_____

# What About Me?

"Do not love the world or anything in the world. If anyone loves the world, the love of the Father is not in him. For everything in the world—the cravings of sinful man, the lust of his eyes and the boasting of what he has and does—comes not from the Father but from the world."
1 John 2:15-16

Okay, I admit it—I love the world. I always have, it's a great place to live. But there was a time when it had me in chains, dying to get out there in it, to live a little. But my situation wouldn't allow it. And God? He never seemed to answer my question, *What about me?* So I decided to put my foot down. One of two things was going to happen: he'd talk to me, or I'd run until I dropped. I had to get his attention...

"Lord, do you hear me?" I took off down the lakeside trail shaking my fist at him as I ran. "Are you listening to me? There's so much I want to see. So many things I want to do. All of my friends are having fun. What about me?"

Silence.

# Answering the Call

"Why won't you answer me? All I ever do is work. I deserve more."

More silence.

"It's not fair!"

I ran until I couldn't take another step, but still God remained silent. Finally I stopped in the middle of the trail and doubled-over, dejected and frustrated, sweating and gasping for air. Physically and emotionally I felt drained. Spiritually I was spent.

"Oh, God," I cried, tears flooding my eyes. "Where are you?"

A funny croaking sound answered me. I turned and watched a frog leap into the lake. "Very funny," I muttered. "Is that the best you can do?" Then a deer caught my eye. She lifted her head from the water's edge, glanced at me and trotted into the woods. "Hmm." A fish jumped and landed with a splash. "What is this?" I murmured. And then I noticed this dragonfly. Crazy thing buzzed past my face, landed on a small branch less than three feet away, and sat there staring at me. I felt puzzled. Was someone trying to tell me something?

Then a high-pitched mechanical sound caught my attention. Distracted I looked up. A fancy motorboat zoomed across the lake. I glanced back at the dragonfly. It sat perched on the end of the stem watching me. I felt a strange awakening in my heart. Then another boat cruised past.

# Answering the Call

My face hardened again. I wanted a boat so bad I could taste it. I balled up my fist and opened my mouth to yell at God, but something stopped me—His voice. It came to me, powerful and resounding, and yet as gentle as a whisper:

*You listen to me now. This world...all those things you so desperately want and can't get your hands on...don't you see? You love those things more than you love me.*

My problems were still waiting for me when I got home, but something about me had changed. I ran into the woods that morning angry, frustrated and shaking my fist at God, but I walked out at peace, quietly acknowledging Him and thanking Him for my life.

Do you ever shake your fist at God? Demand your rights? Then maybe you love this world just a little too much. Put your foot down. Run out there and find Him. And when some silly bug lands on a branch in front of you and boldly stares you down, close your mouth and listen for God's voice. Then follow Him out of that deep, dark forest. He has a better life waiting for you...a life of contentment, of hope, and of joy.

## PRAYER

"Heavenly Father, the cares of this world continually bring me down. Help me to stand tall today, to resist temptation, and to run a good race."

## **APPLICATION**

What is it that you cling to just a little too much? Your rights? Another person? A lifelong dream? Make a short list of the concerns in your life that would seem to tempt you most.

Read 1 John 2:15-16. Into what three categories does the Apostle Paul place the things of this world?

Now take the concerns you listed above and place each one in the appropriate category.

What impact do these concerns have on your daily life? On your relationship with God?

Now read Romans 12:2. What did Paul say would happen if you choose to no longer conform to the patterns of this world?

# BUILDING BLOCKS OF FAITH

Contentment, hope and joy are mine when I walk by
my Savior's side.

## JOURNAL

_____

_____

_____

_____

_____

_____

_____

_____

_____

_____

_____

_____

_____

_____

_____

_____

# I've Realized My Calling

*"I urge you to live a life worthy of the calling you have received. Be completely humble and gentle; be patient, bearing with one another in love."*
Ephesians 4:1-2

"How old is she?" I asked.

"A hundred and one next month. Here's her DNR."

The nurse handed me a piece of yellow paper. I took it and studied it. It bore the familiar red "STOP" sign and the bold command: Do <u>Not</u> Resuscitate! It had been signed by a licensed physician and was well within date. I nodded. There was nothing I could do for the patient anyway.

She lay in the nursing home bed, unresponsive. Each guppy-like breath appeared to be her last. I touched her wrist. It felt warm. A weak pulse tapped beneath the dry, papery skin. I knew it was just a matter of time before it stopped. I glanced at her face. Her eyes looked empty, fixed and drained of life.

"Thank you," I said to the nurse. "We'll take good care of her."

# Answering the Call

I heard sniffles as we loaded the patient onto our stretcher, muted sobs as we rolled her to the ambulance. "Goodbye," a voice said. "We love you, Hattie."

I felt a rainbow of emotions as we pulled away from the scene—sadness, wonder, guilt. The old lady's time had come and there was nothing I could do. But as I sat and watched her respirations slip away it occurred to me that I was witnessing something special, something many people never have a chance to experience—the final moments of another person's life. *What a privilege to be there, I thought, alone with Hattie in the back of my truck.* It was as if I had been invited into the inner sanctuary of something divine.

I felt a sudden yearning to reach out to her, to hold her hand and whisper in her ear. And I knew what I wanted to say. But I wondered, **can she still hear me?** They say hearing is the last sense to go.

I felt guilty as I considered what to do. Who was I to take advantage of her? She was dying. She couldn't possibly defend herself. But what if no one had ever told her? What if she had never heard the truth? This could be her only chance to hear it. It would certainly be her last.

I made my decision.

"Hattie," I said, whispering in her ear. "Can you can hear me? I just want you to know that you're not alone." I squeezed her hand. "Jesus loves you. He's with you now."

# Answering the Call

To my amazement I saw a small tear well up in the corner of her eye. It rolled down her wrinkled cheek and dripped onto the folds of the pillowcase.

Does someone need you? A depressed friend or co-worker? A sister or brother who has long been on your mind? Perhaps all they need is a friend. Someone to stand by their side for that next big step in life.

Hattie didn't die en route to the hospital. We made it to the ER where she lived another forty-five minutes, clinging to life, fighting for every breath until her lungs finally gave out and the cardiac monitor traced a clean flat line. Her life ended peacefully. No advanced procedures. No heroic acts. It was a quiet death. A simple one. And I stayed with her until the end.

The paramedic's job is rarely peaceful. Almost never quiet. So for me, Hattie's passage was a special moment. I even felt as if I'd been invited to be there, to witness the final breath of another human being, a final shallow inspiration followed by a whispery, drawn out, never to be replaced breath of air. What a profound privilege, for it was at that moment I realized my true calling: to be humble and gentle, to serve others during times of greatest need, and to know without question that it's never too late, or wrong, to mention the name, Jesus.

## PRAYER

"Father, help me to live in a manner worthy of my high calling, to be a humble and gentle servant, to love others and to bear their burdens whatever they may be."

# APPLICATION

Do you feel that God created you for a purpose? What do you believe He called you to do with your life?

Are you living a life worthy of that calling?

Reread Ephesians 4:1-2. How are you instructed to live your life? What qualities must you strive to obtain?

Now read Colossians 3:17. What does this passage tell you to do regardless of your calling?

List several steps you will now take to insure you that you live a life worthy of your calling.

# BUILDING BLOCKS OF FAITH

A Christian must clothe himself with humility, gentleness and patience, bearing with other believers, for this is the will of God.

## JOURNAL

_____

_____

_____

_____

_____

_____

_____

_____

_____

_____

_____

_____

_____

_____

# We Must Walk By Faith!

"We live by faith, not by sight."
II Corinthians 5:7

I found the bus parked on the side of the road. A small crowd stood to one side, shocked expressions on their faces. I climbed aboard and found my patient sitting in the aisle on a pile of broken glass, her hands pressed to her forehead, arms and lap stained with blood. She might have been angry—cursing and shaking her fist at the foolhardy teenagers whom had reportedly heaved a rock at the bus, shattering the window and hitting her in the head. But she didn't seem upset.

She took a deep breath, told me her name, and then quietly submitted as I lowered her hands to examine the wound. And it was deep—a three inch gash above her right eyebrow. A golf ball sized hematoma had already formed. Her eyelid looked swollen, discolored and wet.

"It could be worse," I said, taking a wad of water soaked gauze and gently cleansing the site. "But you're going to need stitches."

# Answering the Call

"There's glass in my eye," she said. "I can't open it."

"Don't try."

I finished washing the wound and dressed it with fresh gauze, careful to cover both of her eyes to prevent unintentional movement.

"Now," I said taking her hands, "stand up and follow me. My partner has the stretcher at the bottom of the steps."

I saw her face draw up tight. "But I can't see. How can I—"

"Lisa. Trust me."

"But—"

"Think of it as a faith walk."

Her face relaxed. She nodded as if she understood the meaning of the scripture…to walk by faith means a willingness to close one's eyes. To trust in the Lord, with all of one's heart.

I helped her stand and then backed down the aisle, coaxing her with quiet words of encouragement. Her first few steps seemed timid, unsure, but her faith seemed to grow as we gained momentum. Together we walked down the steps, through the door, and outside into the humid night air.

# Answering the Call

The back of the ambulance was cool and bright. I checked her vital signs and started an IV. We made small talk about the event, about her wounds, and eventually the conversation turned to faith.

"You're a Christian, aren't you?" she said. It was more of a statement than a question.

"Yes, I am."

"Will you pray for me?"

Now I wish I could say I'm a saint, but I'm not. And I wish I could tell you I pray with every patient in the back of my ambulance, but I don't. I've argued with many, fought with a few, and battled my own prejudices more times than I can remember. "But her question? It reminded me...I had a job to do."

"Of course I'll pray with you," I said.

So we prayed. Two people from different worlds meeting in the most unlikely of circumstances, holding hands and praying as if we'd known each other for years. They say God works in strange ways; I see it more as creative brilliance. His love breaks down barriers, shatters human defenses. It brings people together who might otherwise never meet.

"You know what's fascinating?" I said when I raised my head from prayer. "You haven't even seen me yet and still, you trust me."

# Answering the Call

She nodded. Then smiled. I couldn't see beneath the bloody bandages, but I'm sure her eyes twinkled.

"We live by faith," she murmured, "not by sight."

Amen to that.

Are you facing a challenge? A wall too high to climb? Tell the Lord. Trust Him. And then take hold of His gentle hands and follow Him toward the light.

## PRAYER

"Lord, help me to follow you, to trust you with all of my heart, and to walk by faith instead of relying on my own limited judgment."

# APPLICATION

The First Responders in your community—the paramedics, the police officers and firefighters—share a fraternal faith, a trust that is best described as 'watching the other man's back.' They must, for it's a necessary part of the job. But in everyday life it can be difficult to find another person you trust with all you have. Can you describe a situation where you were compelled to trust another person with something precious, like say your life, or that of a family member or close friend?

How did it make you feel to know that one of your most valuable possessions was in another person's hands?

Read Deuteronomy 31:6 and Joshua 1:5. What do these scriptures say regarding God's intention to always watch your back?

How might these promises change your daily life? Your commitment to prayer?

# BUILDING BLOCKS OF FAITH

Trust the Lord, acknowledge Him in all you do, and He
will show you which path to walk.

## JOURNAL

_____

_____

_____

_____

_____

_____

_____

_____

_____

_____

_____

_____

_____

# Clear in Any Language

Finally, all of you, live in harmony with one another; be sympathetic, love as brothers, be compassionate and humble.
1 Peter 3:8

I admit it. I didn't want to touch the guy. He sat on the edge of the bed with his leg elevated. His knee looked swollen and red with infection. Yellow pus oozed from between the stitches. My nose drew up. I felt my guts tighten. I swallowed the bile in the back of my throat and approached him.

"Hey," I said, certain I knew the answer he would give. "Do you speak English?"

He shook his head. I saw fear in his eyes.

I should have introduced myself, made an attempt at friendliness and tried to gain his trust, but I didn't. I performed a rough assessment careful to keep my gloved hands as far away from the festering wound as possible.

# Answering the Call

After checking his vital signs I sent my partner to the truck for the stretcher and quickly wrapped the wound with dressings. I just wanted to get the job done. Get out. Get on to something else. *After all,* I thought, *this guy doesn't deserve my help.* He's just like all the rest of them. He's using us. Trespassing. He doesn't belong here!

My patient seemed to read my mind. He murmured something and tried to stand, but he didn't get far. He grimaced. His red-rimmed eyes filled with tears. He fell back onto the dirty sheets and squeezed his thigh, crying. I couldn't understand what he said but it didn't matter. The pain on his face would have been clear in any language. He needed help.

Suddenly it occurred to me how selfish I had been. I wasn't acting like a Christian at all. There was no kindness in my voice, not a trace of compassion in my touch. I paused and stared deep into his panicked eyes and instantly my vision cleared. No longer was I dealing with an illegal alien. I was helping my fellow man. He had a handsome face and strong brown eyes. He probably even had a proud name.

"My God," I whispered, "forgive me."

I felt new warmth flow through me. I felt stronger, more compassionate. I slowed down, properly dressed his wound, and then stopped and looked him in the eyes.

"Amigo—" I tapped my chest. Shook my head. "I'm sorry, friend. My name is Pat."

# Answering the Call

His eyes widened. The corners of his mouth drew up in a timid smile. "Si," he said. A gentle nod. "Me llamo German…" *(my name is Hermaan)*

We had a short ride to the ER. I rechecked his wound, started an IV, and then sat back and continued my feeble attempt at communication. I stuttered a little, shrugged a lot, and occasionally shook my head. A couple of times I even laughed. So did Hermaan. He still hurt—I could tell by the way he clinched his teeth every time the ambulance hit a bump—but his fear and distrust had vanished.

As we arrived at the hospital it occurred to me that my patient and I had hit it off. He still smelled, his wound still reeked and his clothes still stank, but I no longer cared. I'd made a new friend, and in doing so healed a lifetime of bitterness and distrust.

## PRAYER

"Lord, thank you for loving me. Help me to be kind and compassionate, and to always love my fellow man regardless of his background or race."

# Answering the Call

## APPLICATION

If you are like most people, you struggle with a certain amount of prejudice. Will you be honest with yourself and admit a prejudice you hold toward another race or group of people?


Have you ever been forced to deal with that prejudice through direct encounter with another individual? If so, how did you feel at the time? Superior to the other person? Inferior? Did you experience a certain amount of distrust?


Reread the scripture passage again, I Peter 3:8. How does God expect you to treat that individual?


Now read Ephesians 4:32 to 5:2. Whom do the scriptures say you should imitate whenever you deal with other people? How are you supposed to do it?


What exactly does this passage indicate that Jesus Christ did for you? How might this knowledge change your prejudice toward that person or group of people?

# BUILDING BLOCKS OF FAITH

The fruit of the Holy Spirit are love, joy, peace, patience,
goodness, kindness, faithfulness, gentleness and self-control.

## JOURNAL

_____

_____

_____

_____

_____

_____

_____

_____

_____

_____

_____

_____

_____

_____

_____

_____

# Fight for Position.  Fight!

The LORD is my shepherd; I shall not want.  He ma-
keth me to lie down in green pastures: He leadeth me
beside the still waters.  He restoreth my soul.
Psalm 23:1-3

Total loyalty. Total trust. Total dependence.

Every time I read Psalm 23 I imagine a flock of sheep
fighting for position. They push, they struggle, each trying
his best to draw close to the shepherd's leg while an army
of angry red eyes glares at them from the darkness. They
hear vicious growling, angry pawing, and the relentless
snarling of hungry creatures eager to tear at their soft pink
flesh. But the flock remains safe. It grazes in perfect peace,
totally aware of the dangers, but secure in the knowledge
that the shepherd is keeping watch, his rod and staff in
hand.

What a beautiful image.  No scripture encourages me
more. But when I realize that it was written for me, about
me, I'm humbled.  For I am one of those lost sheep. We
are his flock.

# Answering the Call

We live in a dangerous world, surrounded by terror. Evil men plot against us, to maim, kill, and destroy our way of life. Follow the world, stray off of God's chosen path, and, in the end, you will be dragged down a road of destruction with the eternal darkness of hell at the end. Yes, death is all around us and it can strike at any moment. So what are we to do? Where is our shepherd? Who will raise his staff to fight on our behalf?

As I reflected on the tragedy of 9/11 this week, that question came to mind. On that terrible day 2,983 of our brothers and sisters felt the wolves' teeth tear into their flesh. Evil attacked. And innocent people died. A cruel picture? You bet it is, but it's one we must never forget. If we learn nothing else from their needless sacrifice, let us learn this: Like sheep, we are all vulnerable. We need a shepherd. We need salvation from this lost and dying world.

None of us knows when our time will come, so before you go to work, to class or to bed, ask the Lord Jesus Christ to walk into your life. He is the Great Shepherd, your rock and your fortress against the dangers of this world.

And when the darkness closes in, when the killing wolves attack, draw as close to Him as you can. Fight for position. Fight! And when your time comes—when it's your turn to walk through the Valley of the Shadow of Death—your shepherd will be standing by your side. His rod and his staff, they will protect you!

## PRAYER

The people who went to work that tragic morning, and all of the firefighters, police officers and  paramedics who died in the line of duty, none of them realized their lives would be demanded of them that day.  Help us to learn from their misfortune, to be aware of the dangers surrounding us, and to draw as close to you as we can.  None of us knows when our time will come.

# APPLICATION

Do you remember how you felt on the morning of
9/11/2001 when America fell under attack? Did you
feel frightened? Uncertain? Could you sense the hungry
wolves staring at you from the darkness? Describe the
way you felt that morning.


Read Psalm 23...Try to envision the scene. Can you see
the meadow? The cool blue waters? Can you imagine the
sheep gathered around the shepherd, terrified, fighting
for position to draw as close to his legs as possible as the
fiery red eyes peer at them from the darkness? And the
shepherd? His strong hand tightly gripping his wooden
staff, no trace of fear on his face. Do the sheep appear
safe by his side? Describe how this passage makes you
feel.


Now imagine that you are one of those sheep. How
would you feel if the shepherd suddenly abandoned you
leaving you alone to face the hungry wolves?

# Answering the Call

Read Deuteronomy 31:1-6. What did Moses promise the Israelites regarding the Lord their God?




Now read Joshua 1:1-5. What was God's promise to Joshua?




Also read Matthew 28:16-20. How long did Jesus promise that He would stay with His disciples?




Jesus is the good shepherd (John 10:11). If you are following him you have nothing to fear. How might this change the way you respond the next time you feel frightened?




## BUILDING BLOCKS OF FAITH

God knows the day, the hour, the exact moment your life will end. And after that comes eternity. Do you know Jesus? Have you received His gift of everlasting life?

# Answering the Call

## JOURNAL

_____

_____

_____

_____

_____

_____

_____

_____

_____

_____

_____

_____

_____

_____

_____

_____

_____

_____

# A Real Miracle

*He performs wonders that cannot be fathomed,
miracles that cannot be counted.
Job 5:9*

My job is unpredictable, out of control at times, and just occasionally I need a little help. But sometimes I need a real miracle. My last call was one of those times.

"Excuse me. Move please. Hey! I said, move!"

My partner, Larry, pushed through the crowd of nervous onlookers. He carried an orange airway bag over his shoulder; I carried a ton of uncertainty in my heart. Three men dressed in bunker pants and navy blue fire department tee shirts knelt over a small inert body in the middle of the street. Fire Captain David Young looked up at me and grimaced. "Boy, am I glad to see you guys. His airway's as tight as a plugged pipe."

"How long has he been down?" I asked, glancing at the child's face. The small brown eyes appeared lifeless, the lips the color of a purple Popsicle.

"Six or eight minutes," Young responded. "Maybe more." I sighed, kneeling beside my patient. Larry handed me a bag-valve-mask resuscitator. I placed it over the boy's mouth and nose and gave the bag a squeeze. I hoped to see his chest rise as his tiny lungs filled with air, but it didn't. The air squeaked out of the sides of the mask instead of flowing down his throat and into his lungs. His airway was blocked.

Larry handed me a laryngoscope. I inserted the tip of the blade into the child's mouth and lifted his tongue. The fiber-optic bulb lit the back of his throat all the way to the vocal cords. "Hmm," I murmured. "Not good."

"What is it," Larry said. "See anything?"

"Something's blocking his airway, but I can't see it. Quick," I said, holding out my hand and snapping my fingers. "Let's tube him." Larry placed a clear, slender endotracheal tube into my hand. I inserted it into the boy's throat and passed the tip through the vocal cords, but it stopped short as if hitting a wall. "Something's down there," I said withdrawing the tube, "but I don't see it. Do some more thrusts."

Nobody moved.

"Come on," I shouted. "Do it!"

One of the firefighters straddled the child, placed his hands on the boy's abdomen, and gave five, quick upward thrusts. I tried again. The tube stopped short. I felt myself begin to panic. The child's airway was completely blocked. He was *going* to die. I needed a miracle.

# Answering the Call

What does that scripture say? He performs wonders no man can understand? Miracles too numerous to count?

"Jesus," I whispered. "Help me."

I tried again. No luck. My heart broke.

"Let's go!"

I picked up the boy and ran for the ambulance. I climbed into the back of the truck and placed him on the stretcher. Larry climbed in behind me and slammed the doors. The truck began to move. The siren wailed. We tried again to clear the little boy's airway, first using the Heimlich maneuver, then another ET tube. No change. There was nothing more we could do.

"Oh, Lord," I cried, "Please help us!"

Suddenly I felt a heavy jolt as the truck hit a deep pothole. The rear end jumped up then landed hard on one side and lurched upward again. I lost my balance and fell to the floor. I wanted to curse, to shout out in anger and frustration. *Why did you fail me, God? Why?*

"Hey," Larry shouted. "There it is!"

He reached into the boy's mouth and removed a small round object. He wiped away a layer of creamy white saliva and held it up for me to see.

"It's a grape!"

# Answering the Call

Do you believe in miracles? I sure do. That little boy choked on that grape and should have died. Fifteen minutes without air and life as we know it is all but impossible…but not with God. By the time we left the ER the boy was wide-awake and sitting up with his family, as healthy looking a child as I had ever seen. Yes, I believe in miracles. Our God is real.

Don't you ever give up! No matter how huge the mountain you face, God is bigger. And He still performs wonders, the likes of which no man could ever imagine.

## PRAYER

"Lord, my life is unpredictable. Sometimes out of control. Help me to remember that you are still in charge, always ready to handle even my toughest problems."

# Answering the Call
## APPLICATION

Have you ever been in a situation where you felt totally out of control? When there was nothing left to do but cry for help? Describe that situation.


How did you handle it? Did you pray? Curse? Ask another person for help?


Read Mark 4:35-41. What did Jesus do when his disciples cried out to him for help?


Now read Matthew 14:23-32. What did Jesus do when Peter began to sink?


According to Job 5:9, what kind of wonders does God perform?


Next time you find yourself out of control, how will you respond differently than the previous time?

Answering the Call

# BUILDING BLOCKS OF FAITH
He performs wonders that cannot be fathomed.

## JOURNAL

_____

_____

_____

_____

_____

_____

_____

_____

_____

_____

_____

_____

_____

_____

# A Second Chance

Jesus said to her, "I am the resurrection and the life.
He who believes in me will live, even though he dies; and
whoever lives and believes in me will never die.
Do you believe this?"
John 11:25

I thought I'd been had. A group of old men sat in rocking chairs on the front porch of the retirement home. Their aged faces reflected serenity. Their expressions revealed not a care in the world. I stepped onto the porch and cleared my throat. No one spoke or greeted me. They hardly seemed to notice me.

"Excuse me," I said feeling somewhat confused, quite certain that my EMS uniform would have been enough to announce the purpose of my visit. "Did you gentlemen call 9-1-1?"

"Sure, sure," one of the men said. "We called you."

"Well?" I said with a chuckle. "What can we do for you, sir?"

# Answering the Call

"I think Harold's dead." He pointed across the porch. "Stopped breathing a few minutes ago."

"What?" I hurried over to check Harold's status. Sure enough, the gray-haired old man sat motionless in his rocker, his head slumped against the shoulder of one of his buddies as if asleep. I saw no sign of life, no movement at all. I touched his neck and felt for a pulse. Nothing.

"Uh, Andy?" I glanced at my partner. "I believe he's right."

There's one thing for sure—death awaits us all. But what comes after that? Eternal life? Hell? Nothing? Jesus said whoever believes in Him would live and never die.

Andy powered up the defibrillator unit. I grabbed the old man by the arms, slid him to the floor and ripped open the front of his shirt. Buttons flew. Fabric tore. Andy handed me the paddles. I placed them on his chest. I glanced at the monitor. A squiggly green line traced across the screen.

"Okay, we've got V-Fib," I said. "We can handle that."

Andy switched the unit to DEFIB and pushed the charge button. The unit began to whine. The low-toned whistle built quickly into a high-pitched shrill.

"Okay," Andy said, the capacitor fully charged. "Light him up."

"Clear!"

# Answering the Call

Andy backed away. I straightened my arms, pushed the paddles firmly against Harold's bony chest, and delivered the shock. Two hundred watt-seconds of electricity discharged into the old man's body. His back arched. His muscles jerked. And then suddenly, to my amazement, he opened his eyes. He looked about briefly as if trying to gain his bearings, and then turned and gazed at me.

"Who are you?"

"Sir," I said, trying to hide my astonishment. "I'm a paramedic."

"What are you doing?"

"You were dead, Harold," one of the old men shouted. "These boys saved your life."

"They did? Well, ain't that something?" Harold sat up and rubbed his chin. "Thanks, fellas. Looks like I got me a second chance."

God has offered you a second chance too. A priceless gift called everlasting life. Have you accepted it? Will you?

Harold died that cool autumn evening but apparently God wasn't finished with him. He sent Andy and me, and by the delivery of a single shock of electricity He gave Harold a second shot at life. You may not be as fortunate as Harold was, so don't delay that decision. Say yes to God's Son, Jesus Christ. He is your second chance.

## PRAYER

"Thank you, Heavenly Father, for gift of
everlasting life, and for using Harold to remind me
of the importance of telling others."

# Answering the Call
## APPLICATION

In Ecclesiastes 3:1, King Solomon wrote, "There is a time for everything, and a season for every activity under heaven..." Read verses 2-8. What does this passage tell you about death?

Death is inevitable. The question then is what happens next? The Prophet Daniel wrote, "everyone whose name is found written in the book will be delivered. Multitudes who sleep in the dust of the earth will awake: some to everlasting life, others to shame and everlasting contempt." (See Daniel 12:1-2). If you could choose between the two, would you choose everlasting life or everlasting contempt?

# Answering the Call

Read Romans 6:23. According to this verse what is God's free gift to you?

Now read Romans 10: 9-13. What must a person do in order to receive this free gift?

You do not know when your time will come, but you can experience everlasting life. Will you now accept God's free gift of everlasting life through Jesus Christ?

# BUILDING BLOCKS OF FAITH

Be vigilant. Keep watch. No man knows when his hour
will come.

## JOURNAL

_____

_____

_____

_____

_____

_____

_____

_____

_____

_____

_____

_____

_____

# Power for the Weak

Do you not know? Have you not heard? The LORD
is the everlasting God, the Creator of the ends of the
earth. He will not grow tired or weary, and His understanding no one can fathom. He gives strength to the
weary and increases the power of the weak.
Isaiah 40:28-29

My youngest son was fourteen at the time, healthy, safe,
and getting himself ready for school when my final call of
the night shift began.

"EMS report for medic-seven," the dispatcher said.
"Possible suicide."

Terrible images flooded my mind as I ran for my truck.
Slashed wrists. Gunshot wounds. Horrific expressions of
self-inflicted death.

"You can handle this," I told myself. "It's just another call."

But it wasn't. We found her lying at the base of a carpeted
staircase—a fourteen-year-old girl with no sign of life.

Her eyes bulged. Her face looked puffy and blue. A collar
of swollen red skin encircled her neck.

# Answering the Call

"She hung herself," a police officer explained. "Her little sister found her. Cut her down and ran back to bed. Can you believe it? Poor kid didn't know what else to do."

Have you ever felt the harshness of life slap you in the face? Witnessed death or cruelty, or shared in the suffering of a loved one or friend?

I wanted to cry but I couldn't. My defense mechanisms worked too well. I glanced around the room. Other faces reflected anger, pain and disbelief, but I felt nothing. No sorrow. No pity. Just numbness.

"You can handle it," I whispered. "It's just another call."

Weeks passed, then months. My life went on as usual. Then one day another crisis jolted me, this time in *my* home. I'd lost someone I loved, and I didn't know what to do.

My defense mechanisms went to work again. I prepared myself for the worst.

"You can handle it," I told myself. "It's just another call."

But this time I was wrong. Like a pressure cooker blowing off steam, I exploded. I broke down in a fit of uncontrolled grief while my wife, my sons and my in-laws watched, bewildered by my sudden burst of emotion.

Embarrassment could not begin to explain the humiliation I felt that day. But I couldn't help myself, it just happened. Fifteen years of pent up frustration and anger, grief and hopelessness, sorrow and death—they all finally surfaced, and with them a tidal wave of emotion that truly rocked my world. And for the first time in my life I understood the meaning of the scripture: *He gives strength to the weary and increases the power of the weak.*

"Give me strength, Lord, I'm weary. Give me power, I'm so weak."

My family survived that crisis. God poured out His mercy on us...especially on me. I still find myself crying at times when the harsh realities of life slap me in the face, but I handle the pain better now. I'm stronger, more resilient, better equipped to let it all go.

When you feel tired and weary, unable to manage the stress in your life, ask God for the strength to make it through. The power to push on when you feel you've reached your end.

## PRAYER

"Lord, you have shown me that I can't make it own my own. Thank you for giving me new strength, and for helping me day by day."

## Answering the Call

# APPLICATION

When facing the trials of life it is often difficult to remain focused, to hold one's head high and trust God with all of your heart. Describe a situation where you found yourself overwhelmed, unable to cope with a problem or insurmountable task.

Did you feel stronger because of the challenge or tired and weary due to your lack of situational control?

Did your emotions get the better of you? How did you feel? Frightened? Discouraged? Take a moment to describe your feelings at that moment.

Read Isaiah 40:28-29. What does this passage mean to you? Who provides strength to the weary? Power to the weak?

Answering the Call

Now read Psalm 90:2. What does the Psalm tell you about God?

Also read Isaiah 40:26. Why is it that not a single star is missing? Go outside and study the sky at twilight. Watch the stars appear one by one as the sky turns black. Who is it that Isaiah tells us watches over this event every night?

Next time you feel tired or weary what will you do differently? Remember, God gives strength to the weary and increases the power of the weak.

## BUILDING BLOCKS OF FAITH

God's people shall run and not grow weary. They shall walk and not faint. He gives strength to the weary and power to His saints.

# Answering the Call

## JOURNAL

_____

_____

_____

_____

_____

_____

_____

_____

_____

_____

_____

_____

_____

_____

_____

_____

_____

_____

# The Armor of God

Finally, be strong in the Lord and in his mighty power. Put on the full armor of God so that you can take your stand against the devil's schemes. For our struggle is not against flesh and blood, but against the rulers, against the authorities, against the powers of this dark world and against the spiritual forces of evil in the heavenly realms.
Ephesians 6:10-12

It's my routine each night as I drive to work: Leave the house, drive north 2.5 miles, and then hang a left. The highway is long and straight, and for fifteen miles I'm alone with my thoughts. I use that time to think. And to pray. "Help me to be a good paramedic. Please don't let me hurt anyone tonight. And, Lord, please help me to be a gentleman."

That night I clocked in at 7:00 p.m. and right away the calls began. Tough calls. The kind that make me wonder why I still do this job? One patient lied to my face, another spit at me. A belligerent female cursed at me, blamed me for her plight in life and then accused me of racism.

# Answering the Call

The hours ticked away; the calls continued to come. Exhausted and weary from the workload, I grew frustrated by the onslaught of personal insults. But I remained in control, presented myself as a gentleman.

Until 4:00 a.m.

The armor of God. It protects us from the unexpected, those difficult moments when our faith is tested most.

I found her vehicle atop a grove of broken pines. Prickly vines tore at my skin as I climbed down the embankment and looked the shattered side window into her car. "Hello," I said, scanning my patient for major injuries. "My name's Pat. What's yours?"

"Get me out of here," she shouted.

"Well we will," I said, "but first tell me, are you breathing okay? Are you hurt?"

"Shut up and get me out here," she shouted. "Now!"

Ever find yourself blindsided, hit by a situation that pushed you over the edge?

I bit my tongue and continued my assessment. Trauma victims sometimes speak irrationally, I knew, and say things they don't mean. But I found no major injuries or any reason for her rude belligerence.

I explained the situation to her as the firefighters approached the car. She continued to fuss as they pulled open her door, continued to gripe as we immobilized her to a spine board and carried her up the hill.

She fought me the whole way to the hospital, pulling at her bindings and yelling for me to cut her loose. I tried to remain patient, continued to help. I even stabilized her on a particularly rough section of road—grabbed her belt and held on tight to keep her from rolling as the truck rocked side to side—but she rejected my act of kindness and turned it into something else.

"Don't you do it," she threatened. "Don't you dare touch me like that!"

"What!" I released her belt. "You're accusing me of abusing **you**?"

I couldn't believe it. How much abuse is a man supposed to take? I'd already been reviled, and spit at, and torn to pieces by a tangle of gnarly thorns, but this? Enough was enough. She started to respond to the question but I would not allow it. "Shut up," I said, pushing away and moving as far from her as the ambulance walls would allow.

"What?" she said. A look of incredulity crossed her face. "What did you say to me?"

*"I SAID, SHUT UP!"*

And she did. She remained as passive as a lamb for the rest of the ride. But not me. I marched into the ER full of rage and left a trail of verbal destruction in my wake. I got in trouble of course. The ER doc threatened to write me up, and my supervisor let me hear about it later, but I couldn't have cared less.

I learned a valuable lesson that night—I must put on the full armor of God *every* time I go to work, in fact, every time I leave my house. For I can't make it in this world without God's protection. And neither can you. You must put on the full armor of God too. Be strong in the Lord. Take up your shield and your sword and be strong in His mighty power.

# PRAYER

Protect me from the enemy. Remind me to put on your full armor every day. Forgive me when I fail, Lord, and help me to be a gentleman regardless of what life throws my way.

## APPLICATION

I was not prepared for that shift. My enemy, the devil, was lurking, using every opportunity to attack and slowly break me down, and he used another person to do it. She pushed me too far and I lost my cool. Describe a time you felt the same way. How did you react?

Read Ephesians 6:10-13. Why is it important for the Christian to put on the full armor of God every day? Who or what is it that we struggle against in life?

Reread verse 13. What will you be able to do once you have put on the full armor of God?

Now read Ephesians 6:14-17. List the six different pieces of spiritual armor that are vital for the successful Christian walk.

God provided everything you need to stand your ground against your enemy. Are you wearing His full armor everyday? What practical steps might you now take to strengthen your daily walk with Christ?

## **BUILDING BLOCKS OF FAITH**

The full armor of God—the belt of truth, the breastplate of righteousness, the helmet of salvation, the shield of faith, the sword of the spirit, and the gospel of Jesus Christ.

# Answering the Call

## JOURNAL

_____

_____

_____

_____

_____

_____

_____

_____

_____

_____

_____

_____

_____

_____

_____

_____

_____

_____

# Couldn't Do It Without You

Just as each of us has one body with many members,
and these members do not all have the same function,
so in Christ we who are many form one body, and
each member belongs to all the others. We have different gifts, according to the grace given us.
Romans 12:4-6

We first responders have it rough. We jump when others call, wallow in their blood, manage life-threatening emergencies and occasionally save lives. I'm proud to serve on the front lines of life, but my pride has its limits. I depend on other people. I could never do this job by myself. No way!

"Pat," Captain David Young shouted as I climbed from the ambulance. "You need to intubate him, dude. He's crashing fast!"

I grabbed my trauma bag and started toward the wreck. It looked bad, a Ford pickup wrapped around a tree, its front end crumpled in upon itself like aluminum foil. A team of firefighters and first responders scurried about the scene. Young knelt in the bed of the truck holding a bandage to the victim's head.

"Bring your suction unit too," he yelled. "He's full of blood!"

I ran back, grabbed the necessary equipment, and then trotted to the scene.

"It ain't good," Young said as I approached. "He was leaning against the tailgate when they hit the tree. Flew into the back of the cab headfirst." Young pulled away the trauma dressing. Blood poured from a gash in the center of the victim's head. He quickly recovered the wound and applied direct pressure. "Like I said, not good."

I gazed at my patient. His eyes looked lifeless. He breathed in short gurgling gasps. Young forced open his jaw. I inserted a hard plastic catheter.

"Okay," I said. "Turn it on."

My partner hit the power switch on the suction unit. A long line of bright red blood coursed up the tube. The catheter sucked and hissed, but I was unable to keep up with the steady stream of blood flowing into his mouth. I felt myself begin to panic.

"We're losing him," I said. "Help me!"

"Tell us what to do," somebody said.

"You two," I said pointing at two of the firefighters. "Get

# Answering the Call

a trauma line set up in the back of the truck. And one of you grab the backboard and stretcher." I handed my partner the catheter. "Here, you suction. I'll intubate."

The church is like that group of rescue workers, a team of believers, each with a different role. We all work together for one common good—to serve the Lord. To save people's lives.

And so, we did our jobs. My partner, the firefighters, the police officers controlling the crowd. We worked as a professional team. We suctioned. We intubated. We dressed the bleeding head wound and immobilized our patient. Then we drove him to the emergency room and left him in the doctors' care. We did everything within our collective power to achieve the impossible, to sustain our patient's life, but in my heart I knew he was already gone.

Are you a member of a Church? A group of believers who worship together and pray, each using the gifts he was given to serve the others and to spread the Gospel of the Lord Jesus Christ?

A few years later I transported a young woman to the hospital. She spoke of a bad wreck, of how a pickup truck had slammed into a tree. She'd been driving that evening. Her cousin had been the passenger, leaning against the tailgate when the accident occurred.

"He almost died," she explained. "The impact threw him forward. He hit his head on the cab. He lives on Holloway Street now. He's—"

"Wait a minute," I said interrupting her. "What's your cousin's name?"

She told me.

I felt my eyes widen. "Are you telling me he's alive?"

"Oh, yes," she said. "His fingers still tingle a little, but otherwise he's fine. The paramedics saved him."

It wasn't just the paramedics who saved that man; it was David Young and the other firefighters, the police officers who helped us on the scene, the emergency department staff, the surgical team, and every other physician, nurse and physical therapist involved in his recovery. We worked together as a team, each member performing his or her role for the benefit of the victim, and together we accomplished the impossible.

Just like that special team, we in the church have been called to action. And you have a function. Are you performing it? Join a team of believers and start working for the Body of Christ today.

## PRAYER

God, please bless all the men and women who work
so tirelessly in the field of emergency response.
They make a difference. They save lives. And
sometimes, when we all work together, we can even
accomplish the impossible.

## Answering the Call

# APPLICATION

Teamwork was vital to the success of that EMS call. All members worked together for the common good of the victim, and in the end we succeeded. He survived. Describe a situation where you responded as a member of a team.

What role did you play on the team?

Was the team successful? What would have happened if you had attempted to accomplish the same results alone?

What would have been the result if you had been missing from the team?

Read Romans 12:4-8. What does this passage have to say about the Body of Christ?

## Answering the Call

What function are you providing in the Body of Christ? (Remember the Body is not complete unless every member is performing his/her role.)

## BUILDING BLOCKS OF FAITH

One man's gift is to prophesy. Another's is to serve. One's is to encourage, and another's is to lead. One man's is to teach, and still another's is to show mercy.

Answering the Call

# JOURNAL

_____

_____

_____

_____

_____

_____

_____

_____

_____

_____

_____

_____

_____

_____

_____

_____

_____

_____

# Under His Mighty Wing

He that dwelleth in the secret place of the most
High shall abide under the shadow of the Almighty.
I will say of the LORD, He is my refuge and my for-
tress; my God; in Him I will trust.
Psalm 91:1-2

First Responders deal with potentially dangerous situations
every day. We go on emergency calls that demand a
heightened sense of awareness and a certain amount of
faith in our fellow man. I usually figure that, if I'm careful,
everything will be all right. But you and I know that life
is not always fair. Bad things do happen, even to good
people. So how should we prepare ourselves for the
dangerous moments in life? How can a person ever find
peace knowing that danger could lurk around every
corner?

My father once told me a story of a squadron of WWII
fighter pilots. The commander had his men memorize Psalm
91—a beautiful poem of God's promise of protection, His
angels, and the fortress He provides His people against
the perils of life. Every morning his men stood as a unit
and recited the passage before climbing into their planes

and flying off to fight the Germans. And as the story goes, not one of them was injured during the course of the war. Every man returned safely to his home.

The telling of that story by my father changed my life, for I now understand that God is my fortress. I take comfort in being by his side. Gain strength in knowing He is always there.

"Kim," I called to my wife. "Have you seen Dan?"

"No, I thought he was with you."

I sighed and walked through the house calling my son's name. I was used to it. Dan was a rascal. He was three years old, full of life, and we were late for church.

"Danny," I called. "Where are you, buddy?" Silence. I walked outside and called him again. Nothing. I trotted around the house shouting his name. Still no boy. "Dan?" I yelled. "Where are you?"

I sprinted back to the front of the house. "Kim. He's not here! I can't find him!"

My wife joined me in a frantic search. I felt confused. Desperate. Suddenly I heard a small voice. I ran to the side yard and saw my son walking from our neighbor's house. He had an apple in his hand and a huge smile on his face.

# Answering the Call

I picked up my son and hugged him. I felt frustrated of course, and angry that he'd run off, but he was back home and safe and that was *all* that mattered. We talked about it. It was a short discussion, after all he was only a child, but later my father and I had a much longer chat.

"Son," my dad said, "listen to me. You won't always be there to watch over Dan. He's going to grow up, move out and have his own children, and someday, God forbid, no matter how much you pray for him, something bad *could* happen. That's life. You need to learn to trust the Lord."

That's when he told me the story of the squadron, and how we're to cling to the promises found in Psalm 91. "Do what those pilots did," he said. "Memorize that scripture, recite it every day, and then let Dan go. God will watch over him."

That was over twenty years ago and today Dan and his brother, Phillip, are healthy young men. God did watch over them, and now they are on their own. But, still, not a day goes by that I don't pray those precious words I memorized so long ago. Only now I can rest, for I know my boys are safe and sound, living in the shadow of God's mighty wing.

Do you live in fear? For your life or for that of a loved one? Cling to God's promises. He will help you tackle your fears. And He will walk with you and yours through the darkest valleys of life.

# PRAYER

"Lord, hold my wife, my children, those I love in the palm of your hand. Give your angels charge over them today. Cover them with your feathers that under your mighty wings they might trust."

# Answering the Call

## APPLICATION

Everyone feels frightened from time to time. Describe a moment that you felt truly frightened, for a loved one, or for yourself.


What or whom did you cling to for strength?


Read Psalm 91. God promises a place where you may always find refuge. Where is it?


Who will He send to watch over you during times of need?


"Because he loves me," says the LORD, "I will rescue him." What else does God promise to do for you and your loved ones in this passage?


Would you memorize Psalm 91, and claim its promises every day for the rest of your life? If so, begin now by committing the first two verses to memory. Write the verses here and repeat them throughout the day until they have become engrained in your mind:

# BUILDING BLOCKS OF FAITH

Like a mountain unmoved by the forces of time, The
Lord is my refuge.  My rock.  My salvation.

## JOURNAL

_____

_____

_____

_____

_____

_____

_____

_____

_____

_____

_____

_____

_____

_____

_____

_____

# Created For Good Works

For we are God's workmanship, created in Christ Jesus
to do good works, which God prepared in advance for
us to do.
Ephesians 2:10

Thomas lived in a small group home on the south side of town. He had AIDS, renal failure, high blood pressure, and the night I met him an overall sick feeling he couldn't explain. "I'm due for dialysis tomorrow," he said, "but tonight I just don't feel right."

He didn't look right either. He was only 47, but he looked old and tired as if he'd spent a lifetime on the run, fighting, and struggling just to stay alive.

I wondered what had happened to him. Surely God had created him for a reason, but had he lived a good life? Done the best with what he had? Or had he chosen the wrong path and ended up full of regret?

I performed a quick assessment. Checked his blood pressure and pulse. I hooked up the cardiac monitor and took a look at his heart. Physically he checked out okay, but I sensed something deeper was wrong. I glanced at his face and got the feeling that this was more than just a sick call. He needed to talk to someone. And I was okay with that. "Tell you what," I said. "Let's take a ride."

He smiled and rose to his feet. It was a routine transport. I stuck an 18-gauge IV catheter in his arm, took another look at his EKG, and then leaned back and looked at him as we rode down the highway.

"So, Thomas," I said. "Where are you from?"

"Right here."

"Yeah? Then you remember this place before it became a ghetto."

He nodded.

"Look," I said, "forgive me for prying, but, well, I was just wondering…were you ever in a gang?"

"A gang?" A stern expression tightened his face. "I learned to shoot a gun when I was five years old. Started taking drugs when I was twelve. Did heroin for more than twenty years on the street and then every day in prison for seven more. It won't my mom that taught me all that."

Have you made poor decisions? Feel that you've lost your way? It's not too late to turn around. Jesus is there to help you find your way back.

I gazed at Thomas without speaking. I felt he deserved that.

# Answering the Call

"The alcohol and drugs ruined me. My kidneys are shot now. I don't blame nobody else though. I made the mistakes, and I'll live with 'em. But these gangs you asked about?" He paused and shook his head. "They're bad, man. These kids today will shoot anybody. They steal and rob for drugs. They kill. And those girls? They only keep 'em round for one reason—makin' babies. To the gangs that's all they're good for. My daughter's in one now, you know." He glanced at me as if searching for an answer. "She stays coked up and pregnant most the time."

"Can't you talk to her?" I asked. "Try to help her?"

"No, man, you don't get it. Can't never talk to her no more. Afraid of her. I know it's my fault, she's my child, but that one…she won't created for no good."

I felt a strange paradox as I walked away from the ER: pleased to know that Thomas is a Christian today—he gave his life to Christ somewhere along the way—but saddened by what I had just witnessed: Harsh reality. Not just words from some magazine article about gangs and troubled youth, but real flesh and blood, a grown man who survived the streets only to live and suffer the consequences of his mistakes.

If you've made serious mistakes and feel that you've lost your way, don't surrender. God created you for a reason, to live a good life and to do the best you can with what He gave you. Turn to Him. He loves you. He will help you find your way.

## PRAYER

Lord, help me to remember that I am Your workmanship. Give me the strength to make sound decisions today, and to turn away from the path of sin that eventually leads to death.

# Answering the Call

## APPLICATION

Most likely you have lived what you believe to be a good life. Take a few moments to think about your life. Compose a list of your most important accomplishments.

Do you believe that any of these accomplishments will earn you the right to go to Heaven?

Read Ephesians 2:8-10. What does the scripture say regarding good works?

Why then is it important to live a good life? Read Matthew 5:16, 1 Peter 2:12. According to these verses, what is accomplished as a result of your good works?

Remember salvation is free, but we will all be judged according to the works that we do (See Psalm 9:7-8, and Ecclesiastes 12:13-14). How might this knowledge change your daily life? What steps will you take to glorify your Heavenly Father?

# BUILDING BLOCKS OF FAITH

Doing good works saves no one, but all will be judged
for the works that they do.

## JOURNAL

_____

_____

_____

_____

_____

_____

_____

_____

_____

_____

_____

_____

_____

_____

_____

# Well, what did you expect?

Love your enemies, do good to them, and lend
to them without expecting to get anything back.
Then your reward will be great, and you will be
sons of the Most High, because he is kind to the
ungrateful and wicked.
Luke 6:35

Larry was a junkie. I think he had more toxic chemicals in his veins than blood. I found him lying in the bushes barely breathing, his eyes half-open, pupils like pinpoints. Foamy saliva dripped from the corner of his mouth. Track marks scarred both arms. I knelt beside him, pulled a dirty syringe from his arm, and then opened my med box to prepare a syringe of my own.

"What else do you want?" my partner, Warren, asked me.

"We need an IV."

"You know he's just gonna rip it out, don't you?"

# Answering the Call

I glanced at Larry's face and remembered the last time we'd seen him. The way he'd cussed us out. Treated us with disdain. But then I remembered the scripture…love your enemies. Be kind to others even when you don't expect to receive anything in return.

"Probably," I said, "but let's do it anyway, Warren. Okay?"

"Suit yourself."

Warren shrugged and snatched a 500-cc IV bag from the med box. I wrapped a tourniquet around Larry's arm, thumped up a fat vein, and then jabbed an IV catheter deep into the vessel. The flash chamber filled with blood. I threaded the catheter and attached the IV tubing. Warren set the flow rate to keep the vein open.

Next I selected a small plastic vial and stuck a 3-cc syringe into the round rubbery top. I turned the bottle over, pulled back on the plunger and withdrew two milliliters of clear fluid. After tapping the syringe to clear it of excess air bubbles I attached it to the IV line and pushed the drug into Larry's vein.

Mere seconds passed before his eyes began to flutter. His respirations quickened. He slurped a couple of times as if sucking the remains of a milkshake from a straw and then took a deep breath and sat up. He looked sluggish at first, blurry and unseeing as if covered by a thick haze, but then his constricted pupils dilated and his mental status sharpened to a fine point.

"Hey," I said. "Welcome back."

# Answering the Call

"What happened?"

"You OD'd again," Warren said. "You almost stopped breathing this time, Larry."

I offered Larry my hand to help him up. He slapped it away. "You took away my high, man!" He ripped the IV out of his arm and gave me the finger. Then he stormed off, bleeding from the punctured vein and shouting obscenities at us as he stumbled down the street. I felt stunned. I glanced at my partner.

"Did you see that?"

"Well, what'd you expect?" Warren said. "A thank you note?"

Later I thought about what had happened, about my own highs and lows, and about the many times I've slapped God's hand away when He was trying to help me up. Am I any different than Larry? Are you? You know we all crave the high of lustful living, but in the end that path leads to addiction and death. Christ came to save us from ourselves, to turn us away from the sin that entangles us. So the next time you feel convicted by the helpful words of a friend, don't turn them away. Christ may have sent them to lend you a helping hand.

# PRAYER

Lord, forgive me for the times I may have cursed you, spit in your face, or blamed you for my mistakes. Help me to forgive others when they do the same to me.

# Answering the Call

## APPLICATION

Have you ever been blamed for someone else's mistake? Or rejected or rebuked when you were only trying to help? How did it make you feel? Describe your feelings.


Read John 19:1-18. What does this passage tell us that Pilate and the Roman soldiers did to Jesus Christ?


Read Isaiah 53:5-6 and 1 Peter 2:24-25. Why was it necessary for Christ to suffer this brutal punishment?


Now read Luke 23:34. What did Christ ask the Father to do as He hung upon the cross? Was He speaking only of those present at the time, or was He also speaking of you?


Christ suffered and died so that you might live. He paid the ultimate sacrifice for you. Will you respond differently the next time you are ridiculed, rejected, or unjustly blamed for another's mistake?

# BUILDING BLOCKS OF FAITH

Anyone can love someone back, but to love one's enemies—those who persecute you and revile you and speak harshly about you behind your back—that is the mark of a true Christian.

## JOURNAL

_____

_____

_____

_____

_____

_____

_____

_____

_____

_____

_____

_____

# What's your gift?

Each one should use whatever gift he has received
to serve others, faithfully administering God's
grace in its various forms.
1 Peter 4:10

"How're you doing, brother? Working hard or hardly working?"

My friend, Steve, always greets me that way. It's his trademark and I love it. It usually makes me laugh, helps me prepare for the shift. But I didn't feel much like laughing that night. My heart was heavy. I needed to talk. Steve clocked in and followed me out to the ambulance bay to check the truck.

"So," he said opening the airway bag. "What's bothering you, brother?"

Steve may not have realized it, but at that moment he was doing what the scripture tells us to do, administering God's grace to me. Using his gift of friendship to admonish and build me up. And boy, did I need it.

I shrugged. "I didn't realize it showed."

112

# Answering the Call

"It shows." Steve gave the wrench atop the oxygen bottle a twist. He glanced at the regulator, nodded, and then retightened it and slid the cylinder back into the bag. "You wanna talk?"

"You know that book I've been writing? It was rejected again."

"No way."

"Another publisher said no. But that's not all. This time my agent sent the manuscript back to me. She's giving up on it. Says she can't sell it."

"Hmmm." Steve bit his lip as if trying to hold back a smile. "I probably shouldn't tell you this," he said with a grin, "but deep down, I'm kind of glad."

"Glad?"

"Well, ever since you started writing that book your head's been somewhere else. Your heart's not here anymore, dude. It's like you've already left."

"Steve, I've been writing for over five years. I've worked hard to get published. You don't know how—"

"You've worked hard for this!"

"This? Steve, this job's chewed me up and spit me out so many times I can't think straight anymore. I mean, c'mon, man. We work all the time. We wallow in blood and guts. We go places most people wouldn't get close to. And

# Answering the Call

where's the payoff? When am I ever going to get mine?"

"Is that why you write? To get yours?"

Steve's question hit a raw nerve. It hurt me, because deep inside I knew he was right. God has blessed me so much. How selfish of me to take one of His gifts and use it for personal gain. Are you doing that too? Seeking recognition? Money? Personal pleasure or fame?

"Well," I said with an awkward stammer, "that's not the only reason."

"Look, you may not want to hear this, brother, but I believe God put you here for a reason, and it's not to make money. He's using you in more ways than you know. I mean just think of all the lives you've touched. The people you've saved over the last twenty years. All those students you've trained to be great paramedics. Brother, there are a lot of folks out there who would be much worse off today if not for you. Shoot, a lot of 'em wouldn't even be here."

"So, what am I supposed to do? Just give it all up?"

"No, write. But do it for the right reason. And don't even think about giving up EMS. God's given you a wonderful gift, brother. You need to use it!"

If you're using God's gifts for the wrong reasons then it's time you made a change too. Discover your gifts, then get out there and use them for the right reason—to serve the Lord.

## PRAYER

Heavenly Father, please forgive me for being so selfish.  And thank you for my good friend, Steve.  For using him to remind me how truly blessed I am.  I'm a paramedic, set apart to save lives.  That is my calling.  That is my gift.

# Answering the Call

## APPLICATION

Do you have talents or abilities that set you apart from others? Take a few moments now to create a short list. What are you "good at"?

Read Romans 12:6-8. According to the scripture, how did you acquire these abilities or talents?

Now read Ecclesiastes 9:10. How does God expect you to use these gifts?

Colossians 3:23. For whose glory are you to use your gifts?

According to Galatians 5:19 selfish ambition is just as much a sin as idolatry, drunkenness and sexual immorality. Are you selfishly using the gifts God gave you for your own edification, or are you using them to serve Him?

# BUILDING BLOCKS OF FAITH

There are many kinds of gifts, but there is only one Holy Spirit who freely gives them. A gift is something God expects you to use for His glory. For the edification of the church.

## JOURNAL

_____

_____

_____

_____

_____

_____

_____

_____

_____

_____

_____

_____

_____

_____

# Answering the Call

# Are you ready for this?

Nothing in all creation is hidden from God's sight.
Everything is uncovered and laid bare before the
eyes of him to whom we must give account.
Hebrew 4:13-14

I had just finished writing an EMS report at the hospital
when a fellow paramedic shouted at me from the other
side of the emergency room. "Pat," he said urgency on his
face. "Get over here quick. You need to see this!"

"What is it?"

"Car wreck. Hurry."

I put aside my paperwork and walked across the ER into
Trauma Room-1. A large crowd stood around the gurney.
I didn't find that unusual. That particular ER belongs to
a teaching hospital, so it's quite common to find people
standing around watching the doctors work—stabilizing
critical patients, sewing up flesh, replacing precious blood.
But as we pushed into the room, I sensed something
wrong. The crowd seemed hungry instead of curious,
wide-eyed and full of glee. Their lustful expressions
seemed completely out of place.

118

# Answering the Call

"What's going on?" I asked.

"Are you ready for this?" My co-worker pushed me to the center of the room. "Look."

My eyes flew open wide. A teenaged girl lay on the gurney stripped of all clothing, her figure laid bare for everyone in the room to see. She was about eighteen years old with beautiful blue eyes and long blonde hair. She had a goose egg on the right side of her head. A trace amount of blood stained her cheek and nose. But otherwise she looked unscathed, the victim of a traffic accident that had apparently knocked her out.

I felt stunned. The physicians and nurses were justified in being there, of course. They were the trauma team, they had a job to do. And the removal of clothing is an essential component of the major trauma assessment. Everything must be uncovered to allow for critical judgment of the injuries at hand. But the onlookers? I saw no reason for the rest of the crowd. A dozen men stood there gawking. The poor girl was being violated.

I felt ashamed. I walked out of the room.

I never learned the extent of her injuries, but God used that young woman to teach me a valuable lesson. One day we will all be uncovered, our hearts laid bare before God. And no deed, no thought, no ill-conceived fantasy or spoken word will remain hidden from His view. We will be exposed exactly as we are.

# Answering the Call

Will you be ready when the King of Kings appears? When the Lord God exposes your sins and judges you for all you have done? If you know Jesus Christ you have nothing to fear. His blood covers you, washes you white as snow. But if you don't know Him, eternal judgment awaits, and after that—death. So turn your life over to Jesus Christ today. He is coming back, and when He does there will be no place on Earth to hide.

## PRAYER

"Heavenly Father, I am a sinner. Thank you for sacrificing your Son for me. His shed blood covers my sins. And on the Day of Judgment, as I kneel before your throne, you won't see my filthiness at all. You will see his blood instead."

## APPLICATION

Do you have any secrets? Things that you would prefer no one else ever knew? Well God knows. Psalm 33:15 says He considers everything you do. Read Proverbs 5:21…what does this passage say regarding your actions, your attitudes, your innermost secrets?

Now read Jeremiah 32:17-19. How will God reward you?

Also read Hebrews 4:12-14. List four attributes of God's word and the relevance of these in regard to your secret life.

According to this passage, what aspect of your life is hidden from God's view?

Are you a Christian? Are you living a life of obedience or are you ignoring His commands. Remember, nothing you do, say, or even think is hidden from God.

# BUILDING BLOCKS OF FAITH

God's word penetrates. It divides. It judges the thoughts
and attitudes of the heart.

## JOURNAL

_____

_____

_____

_____

_____

_____

_____

_____

_____

_____

_____

_____

_____

_____

# God Still Knows Exactly What To Do

So do not fear, for I am with you; do not be dismayed, for I am your God. I will strengthen you and help you; I will uphold you with my righteous right hand.
Isaiah 41:10

"I don't know what to do!"

Actress Jennifer Garner spoke that line in the 2001 Academy Award winning film, Pearl Harbor. She starred as Sandra, a young Army nurse serving in a makeshift hospital on Pearl Harbor on the morning of December 7, 1941. Walking wounded arrived by the score, bleeding profusely, their charred and broken bodies beaten to shreds, many with wounds too deep to fix. The doctors, nurses and Army corpsmen did everything they could to manage the unfathomable catastrophe, but the scene was overwhelming. It was too much to manage, too unbelievable to comprehend. Terrified, the young nurse looked around her at the mayhem and cried, "I don't know what to do!"

# Answering the Call

Have you ever been so frightened you didn't know what to do? Well God has the answer. And He promised to provide you strength in those moments, to pick you up and carry you through the darkest hours of your life.

I can only imagine the horrors of that infamous day when our nation came under attack. Bombs fell from the sky. Torpedoes exploded. Over 2,300 brave sailors died and countless more were injured. It was the first time in modern history that we felt the pounding of our enemy's feet on our own soil—this sacred ground, the United States of America—and it angered us! We knew our enemy. We saw the whites of his eyes and the evil of his cause, and in our righteous determination we fought back. And thank God, we won!

But 70 years later we live in a different America. Our moral values have slipped. We've grown politically correct. And the godly principles on which this country was founded no longer seem important. Have we forgotten all that God has done for us?

Well make no mistake—we need Him again. Our world is at war, and just as in 1941 we are the battleground. Only this time we can't see our enemy. We don't know whom to trust. And many Americans have floundered, looking around them at the chaos and crying, "I don't know what to do!"

Well this is still sacred ground. America is still worth fighting for. And God is still in control. So stand up. Remember the Christian principles on which our country was founded. Turn to the one in whom we still trust. And stand your

# Answering the Call

ground. God said, *"Do not fear, for I am with you; do not be dismayed, for I am your God. I will strengthen you and help you; I will uphold you with my righteous right hand."*

So I ask you, as you consider the fate of our great nation— this indivisible union that still provides liberty and justice for all—what are you so worried about? Why are you so afraid? God is still in charge. And if we will humble ourselves, turn back to Him and ask Him to heal our land, in His righteous determination He will do just that. He's still in charge. And He still knows exactly what to do.

## PRAYER

"God, strengthen us now during this most crucial hour. Help us. Hold us in your hand and restore in us the principles that once made this nation great. You are God. You know exactly what to do."

## APPLICATION

Has there ever been a time when you had absolutely no idea what to do? Take a moment and describe the circumstances.

How did you feel at the time? Scared? Confused?

Read Joshua 1:1-9. What encouragement did God give the Israelites three times in this passage?

What promise does this passage provide regarding God's presence in your life?

## BUILDING BLOCKS OF FAITH

If God's people, who are called by His name, will humble themselves, pray, seek His face and turn from their wicked ways, then He will hear from heaven, forgive their sins, and heal their land.

# JOURNAL

_____

_____

_____

_____

_____

_____

_____

_____

_____

_____

_____

_____

_____

_____

_____

_____

_____

# The Best of the Best

Whatever your hand finds to do, do it with all your might.
Ecclesiastes 9:10

To be the **best**: To excel, to outdo all others, to reach a level of accomplishment unsurpassed in one's field. And for a brave young man I know—my good friend's son— it means even more than that. It means to be willing to lay down his life, to sacrifice his freedom that others might live.

"Pat-Man, I need your help. They've called him up again. They're sending my son back over there. I called to ask for your prayers."

As my friend explained the situation I could hear the fear in his voice. I assured him I would pray for his son, and that everything would be all right, but my heart felt heavy as I hung up the phone. His young man had just gotten home, retired from the military and started a bright new career as a firefighter and EMT, and suddenly, without warning, they had decided to call him back. It didn't seem right. Why couldn't they just leave him alone?

# Answering the Call

But deep inside I knew the reason why. It's because he's one of the best shooters in the U.S. Army. One of the elite. The best of the best.

Has God given you a special talent? A unique ability? A particular skill He wants you to use?

I've known many brave 1st responders: police officers and firefighters, EMTs and paramedics. Men and women with tough jobs who work hard to save other lives. But this young soldier has the hardest job of all. Surgical removal. One shot, one kill.

"A sniper! Hey, wait a minute. Pulling a trigger and deliberately killing another man? How can that be right?"

Well the Bible is full of similar stories. Men who were called on to fight, to play a part in God's divine plan. Take King David for instance, a man after God's own heart. As a young boy he attacked and killed the giant Philistine with a sling and a single stone. God called Him to battle and gave him the strength to complete the task. And Samson, a man made strong by God's own hand. The Spirit of the Lord came upon him in power, and he killed a thousand Philistines with the jawbone of a donkey.

Sometimes God uses rough men to accomplish His will. Men who are willing to use the gifts He gave them, to follow orders regardless of the cost. So when I consider this young man's sacrifices, his skills and his God-given talents, I suddenly understand what it means to be the best. It means to do whatsoever your hand finds to do, and to do it with all of your might.

# Answering the Call

Are you doing the best you can with the gifts and talents God gave you? Don't waste another day. Find out what it is God has called you to do, and then do it. He will give you the power you need to succeed.

## PRAYER

"Lord, please tell him how proud I am to know him, how much his sacrifice means, and how much I appreciate his willingness to fight...for my family, for my country, for my home. Honor and bless him, Lord. Grant him the strength to do his job well, and then bring him back home again so that he, too, may enjoy the blessings of liberty for which he has fought."

## APPLICATION

Write a list of the jobs you have had in your life, or some of the important tasks you have been asked to accomplish. Afterwards, read each one aloud and ask yourself the following question—did I do my best?


Read the scripture passage again. What are you commanded to do when you work, whatever the task?


Now read Colossians 3:22-24. When you work, whom do you serve?


And why is it important to work at your job with all of your heart?


## BUILDING BLOCKS OF FAITH

Make wise decisions. Use your time wisely. In the grave where you are going there is no more work. No more planning. No more wisdom. No more knowledge.

# Answering the Call

## JOURNAL

_____

_____

_____

_____

_____

_____

_____

_____

_____

_____

_____

_____

_____

_____

_____

_____

_____

_____

_____

# Rejoice! It's Christmas!

For the wages of sin is death, but the gift of God is
eternal life in Christ Jesus our Lord.
Romans 6:23

Oh, Lord, not now. It's Christmas...

Larry's compressions were perfect. Two inches deep, a hundred a minute, right out of the book. John had the airway under control, an endotracheal tube in place, properly secured and ventilated. My partner, A.J., started the IV and handed me drugs. Epinephrine. Atropine. I pushed them into the IV line, delivering just the right amount to stimulate the old man's heart. In all it was a perfectly run code, an organized attempt to save a human life. It could not have gone any better. But deep inside I knew it was futile, he wasn't going to make it.

"I don't know," I said shaking my head. "This just isn't working. I think it's time to stop." I glanced at A.J. "What do you think?"

"No," a voice behind me said. "Please don't stop! C'mon, daddy," the young woman cried. "You can do it!"

136

# Answering the Call

I glanced around me at my patient's family, a wife and three grown children. Their cries of support, the hope I saw on their faces, it all just about broke my heart. We'd done everything right, run a perfect code in the middle of their living room—a beautiful home decorated with Christmas tree and lights—but a flat green line traced across the ECG screen. It painted a picture of finality, a portrait of hopelessness and death.

"It's Christmas, dad. You can't leave us now!"

"Honey, stay with us," his wife cried. "We need you here."

If there were no sin in the world, there would be no death. But we live in an imperfect world. Everyone sins. We all fall short of God's standard. Therefore death is inevitable. But, oh Lord, sometimes it hurts so much…

I felt my eyes well up. I shook my head. "It's no use. He's already had three rounds of epi and atropine. One of bicarb. Pacemaker won't capture…"

I paused and glanced at the family again. I could feel their pain, sense their loss. But as I considered my protocol I knew what I had to do.

"Larry," I said my heart breaking as I spoke the words, "hold compressions."

I placed my fingertips against the old man's neck. Larry took a much-needed breather. I squinted and stared at the cardiac monitor hoping to detect a sign of life—a blip, a pulse, any indication that my patient's heart had responded to treatment—but the thin green line continued its lonely trek across the screen. My fingers felt nothing but cool dry skin beneath them. No pulse. No warmth. No life.

I glanced at Larry and shook my head.

"You can stop."

I stood and faced the family.

"Folks…"

I took a deep breath. A fist-sized lump threatened to close my throat.

"I'm so sorry."

It's hard to lose a loved one, especially when our thoughts turn homeward and old memories of Christmas fill us with hope and joy, but there's never a convenient time. Death always seems to surprise us. It's so final, and at times seems so unfair. So what's a family to do when they face such terrible loss? Where can they find peace? Where's the hope?

In Christ alone.

If we were totally obedient to God we wouldn't need a savior. But we're not. The Bible says we have all sinned. And with sin comes eternal darkness. But let the world rejoice, for two thousand years ago God sent his son, Jesus Christ, our one and only promise for everlasting life.

## PRAYER

"I was destined to die but you saved me. Thank you for Christmas, for a new beginning, for everlasting life."

# Answering the Call

## APPLICATION

Are you totally obedient to God? Of course not. No one is perfect. James 3:2 reads, "**We all stumble in many ways**." Read Romans 3:23. What does the Bible say we all have in common?




In what areas of your life do you feel that you are being disobedient to God?




Now read Romans 6:23. What will happen to each of us as a result of this failure?




What is God's solution to this problem?




God has offered you the free gift of eternal life? Have you accepted it? If not will you do so today? If you have accepted Christ will you decide today to live a life of obedience? What steps will you now take toward that commitment?

# BUILDING BLOCKS OF FAITH

Jesus Christ: Wonderful Counselor, Mighty God,
Everlasting Father, Prince of Peace.

## JOURNAL

_____

_____

_____

_____

_____

_____

_____

_____

_____

_____

_____

_____

_____

_____

_____

_____

# We Need a Revival!

"For God so loved the world that he gave his one and only Son, that whoever believes in him shall not perish but have eternal life."
John 3:16

Someone needs to tell these kids. They're all gonna die if they keep living like this…

"Medic-7," the station loudspeaker announced. "Got one shot!"

I grabbed my stethoscope and followed my partner to the ambulance wondering what we would find when we arrived on scene this time. Another gang member? Another kid? I had learned to expect almost anything. Our streets had become a ghetto. A cesspool of drugs and crime.

"A teenaged male shot once in the head," the dispatcher continued. "Police officer on the scene requesting Code-3 response. Code-3."

"10-4," my partner responded jumping behind the wheel and keying the mike. "Medic-7 en route."

# Answering the Call

I climbed into the passenger seat and buckled up. I grabbed a pair of latex gloves and pulled one on each hand as my partner pulled into traffic. I tried to calm myself as he hurried to the scene. *Relax. You've been a medic for a long time. You've seen this before.* But as we pulled onto Hopkins Street I felt my stomach tighten. My palms began to sweat. There's just something unsettling about a young man with a bullet hole in the side of his head, his life blood spilling out all over the ground and a dangerous crowd pressing in on you demanding you get to work.

There was nothing we could do of course. But for the sake of our own skins and the fact that we were standing on their turf and outnumbered about a hundred to one, we made a good show of it. We loaded him up and moved to the truck assuring the angry crowd we would do our best to save him. Once clear of the scene, however, my partner killed the lights and sirens and slowed down to normal traffic. I stared into the victim's lifeless eyes trying to guess his age. Eighteen years old, maybe? Nineteen? Oh, Lord, what a waste.

"Duke ER," I said keying the radio mike. "I'm sorry but we're bringing you a corpse. Another gang member got shot. There's nothing we can do."

For that young man, no, there was nothing we could do. But it's not too late to help the others, the kids still out there on our streets. It's time for a revival. Time to take Christ's message of hope to the broken world of our inner cities.

# Answering the Call

Have you witnessed the hopelessness in our society? The violence and pain? Are you doing anything about it?

Let's take our streets captive for Jesus. Take the gospel out there and see what God can do. For God so loved the world that He gave His only son, for these young people, and indeed, for the entire world.

## PRAYER

"Help us retake our city for Christ. I ask for power and protection, for the First Responders who are out there everyday sharing the love of Christ. Give us opportunities to reach those who have no hope, and the courage to risk it all for the Lord. Dear God, we need a revival.

# Answering the Call

## APPLICATION

Our streets are full of people who need to hear the Gospel. But then so are our schools, our neighborhoods, the places we all go to work. Did any person come to mind when you read this devotion? Write down their name.

Describe them—what do they look like? What color are their eyes?

What is it about that person that draws you to them?

Read John 3:16 again. For whom did God send His only son?

Would you be so bold as to pray for this person, and then to go to them to tell them about Jesus Christ? What steps will you now take?

# BUILDING BLOCKS OF FAITH

God's promise is for you, and for your children, for all who are
far off, even as many as the Lord our God shall call.

## JOURNAL

_____

_____

_____

_____

_____

_____

_____

_____

_____

_____

_____

_____

_____

_____

_____

_____

# Coolest of the Cool

Boldly and without hindrance he preached the
kingdom of God and taught about the
Lord Jesus Christ.
Acts 28:31

I couldn't believe it! He was the coolest of the cool, onetime warlord of the most vicious gang that had ever roamed the streets of New York City, and he was coming to town. I had to see him!

I'd read his book. Well, at least part of it. I couldn't get enough of the rumbles, the switchblades, and the blood, but when he started talking about God, I put the book down. I just wasn't interested in hearing about salvation. But what I didn't realize at thirteen years of age was that God **was** interested in me. He had a plan for my life, and it began the day I picked up that book—**Run Baby, Run**.

"Nicky Cruz? He's coming to town?"

Wild with anticipation I put on my denim jacket and boots. I slid a fake switchblade into my pocket and followed my sister downtown. The auditorium was packed. A feeling of intensity gripped the room. And then I saw him step to the podium. I gazed in amazement. He was everything I had imagined and more. Solid. Tough looking and scarred. I couldn't believe I was actually looking at Nicky Cruz.

He spoke of the ghetto, and of zip guns and chains and blood. And the excitement I'd felt when I'd first read his book hit me all over again. But as he shared the rest of his story I felt a deep yearning. Whatever that tough Puerto Rican kid had found after years of fighting and running from God—I wanted it.

"Jesus saved me," Nicky exclaimed, "and he can save you too!"

The service drew to a close. Nicky gave the altar call. I inched forward with a hundred other people. I didn't even know why. But then Nicky prayed and something remarkable happened to me, and since that moment my life has never been the same.

"Did you do it?" my sister asked me at the conclusion of the service. "Did you pray?"

"Nah," I said, coolly shaking my head. "I just wanted to see what he looked like. He was cool!"

But I did do it—I bowed my head that night and prayed to receive Christ. So thank you, Nicky. God used you to ignite a fire in me. I thank God for your boldness. I thank God for you. You are still my hero. The coolest of the cool!

# Answering the Call

Have you met the Lord Jesus? Have you responded to his call? If not, don't waste another day. Get down on your knees right now and invite Christ into your life. Take it from a man who knows—from a naïve teenaged boy who responded almost forty years ago—you'll be glad you did.

## PRAYER

"Thank you, Heavenly Father, for sending Nicky Cruz. Now send me. There are others who need to know. And fill me with that same boldness, Lord. For if Jesus can save Nicky and me, then He can save them too."

# Answering the Call

## APPLICATION

If not for a brave young preacher named David Wilkerson, Nicky Cruz may have never heard about the Lord Jesus Christ. And if not for Nicky, I may have never heard. What about you? Who first told you about Christ? Have you made a decision to follow Him? If not will you do so now?

If you have already given your life to Christ, have you shared your faith with anyone else? Read Hebrews 13:16. Why is it important to share your faith with others?

Read Acts 4:1-20. How did Peter and John respond (v. 20) when ordered by the rulers and elders to stop speaking of or teaching about the Lord Jesus?

Do you share their zeal? If not do you feel that you should?

How different might your life be today if no one had bothered to tell you about Christ? Will you commit to sharing the Gospel of Jesus Christ with someone you know?

# BUILDING BLOCKS OF FAITH

Remember it only takes one spark to ignite a raging fire.

## JOURNAL

_____

_____

_____

_____

_____

_____

_____

_____

_____

_____

_____

_____

_____

_____

_____

_____

# A Child is Born

For unto us a child is born, unto us a son is given;
and the government shall be on his shoulder; and
his name shall be called Wonderful, Counselor, The
mighty God, The everlasting Father,
The Prince of Peace.
Isaiah 9:6 (KJV)

"Hey, I know you!"

I stared at the woman trying to make a connection. She looked vaguely familiar to me, standing in the booking area of the police station with handcuffs about her wrists, but I couldn't place her face.

"You delivered my baby," she said as the arresting officer removed the cuffs. "Six months ago in the elevator? Remember?"

And suddenly I did remember. Oh, how I remembered…

The house was cluttered. Dingy and hot. A drunk, heavyset male lay passed out on the living room floor.

# Answering the Call

She lay by his side in the middle of the room cursing, her knees apart, her swollen belly exposed. "How far along are you?" I asked kneeling to begin my assessment.

"Don't touch me," she shouted. "Take me to the hospital!"

"Relax, I'm going to help you."

"I don't want your help. I want a ride!"

Her face drew up tight. She took a breath and held it. Her cheeks turned red. And then suddenly a loud cry burst forth. She moaned and screamed and panted and cried until the contraction eased. Then she sat there panting, angry and belligerent. And the rest of the call was pretty much the same. She griped and complained all the way to the hospital, fussing about her treatment in life and all of the bad things people had done to her. "They don't understand. I deserve better." And on, and on, and on.

I ignored her vulgar language and pulled together the equipment for a complicated delivery, all the time praying for the baby yet to be born. We backed into the ambulance bay. My partner opened the doors. We wheeled her inside the hospital and entered the elevator that would take us upstairs to Labor & Delivery. Another contraction gripped her. "It's coming," she screamed as the elevator began to rise. "Oh God, it's out!"

I lifted the sheet that covered her and saw a small baby boy lying on the stretcher between her legs—small and blue and slippery looking. And still.

# Answering the Call

I picked him up and quickly toweled him off. Then I suctioned his mouth and nose. I vigorously rubbed his tiny back to stimulate respiration. Finally he gasped and took a shallow breath. I rushed him into Labor & Delivery with my partner pushing the stretcher at my heels. The nurses welcomed us warmly, but as they realized the baby's distressed condition they quickly took over and went to work.

I felt the excitement one can only understand upon having witnessed the arrival of a new life, but my heart could not rejoice. I didn't know if he would survive. And a few moments later, when the doctor told me the mother had confessed to smoking crack that night, I became almost sick. "That poor child," I murmured. "He doesn't have a chance."

He did live, but upon seeing his mother in the booking area of the police department I realized all over again that the poor child had a tough life ahead. I still pray that he makes it.

When I think of this child's birth and the circumstances surrounding his untimely delivery, I am reminded of another poor baby born in a lonely stable in Bethlehem, before hospitals, before medical care. Who would have thought *he* had a chance? But he came. He lived. He died on a cross and rose from the dead to bring hope to a dying world. Without Christ none of us have a chance. But be of good cheer, it's Christmas, and unto you a savior was born—Jesus Christ the Lord.

## PRAYER

Heavenly Father, protect that baby boy. Make him healthy and strong. And one day, when the time is just right, have someone tell him about Jesus. The Everlasting Father. Prince of Peace.

## APPLICATION

Two thousand years ago a baby was born under the worst of conditions. He spent his first night in a crib made of wood and lined with animal fodder. Read the scripture again, Isaiah 9:6…what are some of the names given to that baby boy?

Now continue by reading the next verse, Isaiah 9:7. What does this passage indicate that he will accomplish?

Many people are born under bad conditions. Others live their entire lives struggling simply to survive. But it is never hopeless, for unto us a child was born. Unto us a savior was given. How might this knowledge change the way you think about your current situation? About another person you know?

## BUILDING BLOCKS OF FAITH

Jesus loves the little children, all the little children of the world.

# Answering the Call

## JOURNAL

# Do You Believe This?

Jesus said, "I am the resurrection and the life. He who believes in me will live, even though he dies; and whoever lives and believes in me will never die. Do you believe this?"
John 11:25-26

We call it a Code. Someone else's heart has stopped beating, and our response—how well we manage our crews and our skills and our abilities to hold it all together—can determine whether the victim lives or dies. It's a scenario paramedics and EMT's practice over and over again to perfection. A rapid response followed by a few moments of controlled fury as we feverishly struggle to save another person's life. And sometimes our practice pays off. This time, however, there was nothing my partner and I could do…

"Medic-seven," the dispatcher said, her voice echoing across the ambulance bay. "Cardiac arrest."

My heart skipped a beat.

"A ninety-two year old female," the dispatcher continued. "Not breathing."

# Answering the Call

My partner entered the address into the GPS unit. I hit the gas. We made excellent time weaving through traffic and arrived on scene only four minutes after the dispatch, but it wasn't soon enough. Our patient was already gone. She lay on the floor beside her bed with no sign of life. Her eyes, frosty and opaque, painted a picture of recent death. Her heart was silent. It was easy to see she was gone.

The Bible says that those who believe in Christ will **never** die. That if you call on His name you will live forever. Do you believe this?

I felt sad as we drove back to the station. Another life had ended, and there was nothing I could do about it. I backed the truck into the bay and was just about to climb out of it when we received another call. Another cardiac arrest. Only this time the victim was much younger, only four months old. We found her lying in bed, her tiny limbs stiff and cool, her skin a sickening shade of blue.

I felt my heart break. I glanced at the young family standing on the other side of the room. I wanted to say something to them but couldn't find the words. On the children's faces I saw shocked innocence, on their mother's unimaginable pain. A bright Christmas tree glowed in the corner of the room but it seemed to lack the luster it might have just hours earlier, before death entered their home robbing them of Christmas joy.

# Answering the Call

Have you ever lost a loved one unexpectedly? Felt the sting of death? The realization that there was nothing you could have done to prevent it?

The loss of these two fragile lives should serve as a grim reminder that death is inevitable. No man knows when his time will come. As fish are caught in a cruel net, or birds are caught in a snare, we all fall victim to physical death sooner or later. So consider this: Jesus said, "I am the resurrection and the life. He who believes in me will never die." Physical death will happen, it's true, but the spirit can live on forever. Do you believe this?

Ask Jesus Christ to be your Savior and Lord. Do it today. And if you already know Him introduce Him to someone you love, for no man knows when his hour will come.

## PRAYER

"Heavenly Father, when I witness death I can't help but wonder—did that person know you? Did they accept your gift of everlasting life? Give me the courage to tell another person, Lord. There are so many people who still don't know."

# Answering the Call

## APPLICATION

Have you ever lost a loved one? Do you find yourself wondering where they will spend eternity? The scriptures are clear on this matter. Read John 3:1-7. What does Christ say here regarding the Kingdom of Heaven?

Now read John 1:1-14. Who is "the Word" that John was referring to in verse 1 where he wrote, "In the beginning was the Word, and the Word was with God, and the Word was God"?

Do you believe this? That Christ was here from the beginning and is in fact, God?

Take a look at 1 John 1:9. What must a man do to be born again?

There are many people in your life that do not know where they will spend eternity. Read Matthew 28:16-20. What is your responsibility as a follower of Jesus Christ?

# BUILDING BLOCKS OF FAITH

Live for today, it may be your last day on earth.

## JOURNAL

_____

_____

_____

_____

_____

_____

_____

_____

_____

_____

_____

_____

_____

_____

# Wake Up, Lord. Save Me!

The disciples went and woke him, saying, "Lord, save us! We're going to drown!" He replied, "You of little faith, why are you so afraid?" Then he got up and rebuked the winds and the waves, and it was completely calm."
Matthew 8:25-27

"How long?" I asked. "How long was she under?"

"Five minutes?" the teenager cried. "Maybe more, I don't know!"

I laid my patient on a dry portion of cement beside the pool. The pretty little pig-tailed girl with chubby cheeks and dimples looked to be about eight years old, and as cute as a button, but her lightly freckled face looked dull and colorless, her eyes as lifeless as a plastic baby doll's.

"Is she going to be all right?" her sister exclaimed. "I only took my eye off of her for a minute!"

# Answering the Call

"Quick," I said tearing open the plastic wrapper for an Ambu-bag. "Get the monitor."

My partner grabbed the EKG monitor and removed the electrode cables.

"Somebody start compressions."

I placed the resuscitator unit over the patient's mouth and gave the bag a squeeze. Her chest rose and fell. Water trickled from the corner of her mouth. One of the firefighters removed his helmet and knelt by my side. He placed his hands on her chest and started pushing against her breastbone with a verbal cadence of one, and two, and three...

"Folks," I heard my partner say, "please stand back. Give us room." He pulled the backing off of a sticky electrode pad and attached it to one of her legs. He repeated the process on each of her other limbs while the firefighter and I performed CPR. "Okay," he said turning on the unit. The EKG monitor beeped. A harsh, erratic, jumpy yellow line traced across the screen. "Let's take a look." He placed a hand on the firefighter's arm. "Hold compressions."

The firefighter stopped. I held my breath. The EKG line flattened out, hiccupped once, and then grew into a regular pattern of uniform complexes. *Oh, thank you, Jesus!*

*Why did you ever doubt me?* I heard the Lord say. *If I calm the mighty oceans, I can certainly take care of you.*

# Answering the Call

I felt elated. I gave our patient two more full ventilations, and then I watched in amazement as she began to cough and choke. We rolled her onto her side, careful to protect her head and neck as the clear pool water drained from her mouth and nose. "Here's oxygen," someone said placing a hissing oxygen mask over the little girl's face. I watched and waited, speaking quietly to her and praying silently as I coaxed her back to life. "Come on," I said. "You can do it. Come on back to us, come back."

She opened her eyes. Her skin turned pink. Then, as if waking from a nightmare and realizing it was all just a terrible dream, she closed her innocent blue eyes again and began to cry. I closed mine too, but I began to pray.

"Thank you," I murmured. "Oh, Lord, thank you so much."

Have you been there? Where the cares of this world make you feel like you're about to drown? Well next time you find yourself in the midst of a raging tempest, with the wind shrieking and waves crashing all around, remember you're not alone. Jesus is right there with you ready to calm the raging storms in your life.

## PRAYER

"Lord, I'm struggling. I feel like I'm drowning down here. I can see the surface but I just can't seem to get there. Help me! Give me your hand, Lord. Please save me!"

# Answering the Call

## APPLICATION

Are you troubled? Are there any problems you can't quite seem to manage? Make a list of some of the storms you have been battling recently.

Read Philippians 4:6-7. In this passage the Apostle Paul encourages you not to worry about these problems. What does he suggest you do instead?

Is there a promise attached to these words of encouragement?

Now read 1 Peter 5:7. What does Peter have to say about anxiety?

Are there steps you can take toward a more peaceful life? A life free of fear and anxiety? Describe how you might accomplish this.

# BUILDING BLOCKS OF FAITH

We serve a mighty King. Nothing is too difficult for God.

## JOURNAL

_____

_____

_____

_____

_____

_____

_____

_____

_____

_____

_____

_____

_____

_____

# I Am Not Ashamed!

"For I am not ashamed of the gospel of Christ: for
it is the power of God unto salvation to every one
that believeth; to the Jew first,
and also to the Greek."
Romans 1:16 (KJV)

"Excuse me," I said looking up at the man. He was huge. Powerful. Broad chest and shoulders clothed in a white karate ghi. And he looked every bit the part, a professional fighter with a knack for breaking bones. In fact he had just broken a pile of concrete blocks…with his head. "Um, Mr. Barlow?"

"Yes?" Frank Barlow turned and looked down at me. "I'm in a hurry, son. How can I help you?"

"I, uh, I just wanted to ask you…" I hesitated and then just blurted it out. "Do you know Jesus?"

Mr. Barlow appeared stunned, caught off guard, but then he chuckled and retaliated as a humored smile broke the stiffness on his face. "Son," he said, "I don't have time for religion right now. I have more important things on my mind."

# Answering the Call

I grinned sheepishly. I knew I was licked. Besides I didn't know what to say or do next. For that matter, I had no idea why I'd even asked him the question. It was just something I felt compelled to do.

"Okay," I said. "I really enjoyed your presentation."

Mr. Barlow nodded, smiled at me, and walked away. I never saw him again.

A few months later my mother told me a story. She had been at a gathering of Christian women that day, a lady's luncheon of sorts. "We had a guest speaker," she said. "He was a karate expert."

"Really?" I was enamored with the notion of karate. Of black belts and fists. Of breaking boards and blocks and people's heads with nothing but hands and feet. "Who was it?"

"Frank Barlow."

"What?"

"He gave his testimony," she explained. "About how he'd become a Christian. About how he was on his way back to his car after a karate exhibition when this high school kid came up to him and asked him if he knew Jesus."

"Mama, that was me!"

"I know," my mom said with a smile. "I just thought you might want to know you had an impact on his life. He accepted Christ."

# Answering the Call

The gospel of Christ is powerful. Life changing. And it's meant for people of all nations—Jews and Gentiles. Everyone.

That was thirty-five years ago. For more than twenty of those years Mr. Barlow operated a dojo in my hometown, called "Judo and Karate for Christ." Today he is a Karate Master, with a 6th Dan black belt in Shorin Jiu Te Do Karate and expertise in numerous other disciplines. But today something else is different about him too…today Frank Barlow knows Jesus.

Are you a Christian? Is there someone you know who needs to know the truth? Then tell them about Jesus. If a skinny eighteen year-old kid can turn a powerful karate expert around by asking him a simple question, then imagine what you could do.

## PRAYER

"Lord, if you could use me then, you can use me now. Help me to be as bold today as I was that day. There are plenty of other people out there who still need to know Jesus."

# Answering the Call

## APPLICATION

If you are a First Responder you have frequent opportunities to serve others—to exhibit true concern, to show compassion, and just as important to share your faith in Christ. You see people when they are hurting, seldom at their best. Have you ever felt compelled to share your faith with another person and then failed to do so? Describe a situation where that happened.

Could you feel your pulse increase? Did your hands become clammy and cold? Perhaps you were concerned about how that person might respond, or that someone else might hear you sharing your faith. Describe your emotions at that moment.

Read Mark 8:38. How does Christ say he will respond if you are ashamed of him?

Now read Luke 22:34. What did Christ predict that Simon Peter would do three times before the rooster crowed?

# Answering the Call

Look a little further down at verses 54 to 62. Explain in your own words what happened.

Is someone on your mind right now? Write down their name.

Will you commit to pray for this person and then to boldly ask them if they know Jesus Christ?

## BUILDING BLOCKS OF FAITH
The Lord is my light and my salvation—
whom shall I fear?

# Answering the Call

## JOURNAL

_____

_____

_____

_____

_____

_____

_____

_____

_____

_____

_____

_____

_____

_____

_____

_____

_____

_____

_____

# What Do You Know?

*In the beginning God created the heavens
and the earth…*
Genesis 1:1

"You know, you should look at the Milky Way sometime, Bill. Some night when the sky is pitch black. As your eyes begin to adjust and that soft, almost indistinguishable blanket of stars and interstellar gases begins to form, you'll realize you're looking at something far greater than us. Our galaxy! It's over a hundred and fifty thousand light years across. And it contains over a hundred billion stars. And they say it's just one of a hundred billion similar galaxies that move around the universe together. How can that be? How did it all get here? It didn't just happen. You say you wonder if there's a God; I don't. I know there's a God. There has to be."

My friend, Bill, gazed at me and scratched his chin, his computer mind processing the picture and considering it from every angle. He gave a slight nod and then an almost imperceptible shake of his head.

"You may be right," he said. "I don't know. I just don't know."

# Answering the Call

The child had curly red hair, a pale freckled complexion, and blue eyes that might have sparkled one day, but it wasn't meant to be. It was his time. Fourteen months old and *already* his time.

Why? I don't know.

When my partner and I arrived the firefighters were already performing CPR. The little boy lay on the ground with his tiny chest exposed. One firefighter's hands pushed against his sternum, another's worked an Ambu-bag pumping oxygen into his lungs at a steady, controlled rate. The mother stood to one side with her hands to her mouth and a stunned expression on her face.

"Oh, Jesus," I prayed as I climbed down from the ambulance. "Lord, please help me. Help me do this right."

My partner and I rushed over to help. I performed a quick assessment and attached the cardiac monitor to confirm a rhythm. There wasn't one. A flat green line traced across the screen. I felt my heart sink. I knew the child was already dead, but I also knew we had to try.

"Good job, everyone," I said trying to keep my cool. "You're doing great. Keep doing exactly what you're doing."

I could tell by their faces that everyone else felt exactly as I did. Confused and scared. A tiny life was slipping away right before our eyes. We all knew our attempts were likely futile. But we held ourselves together. We did it right. Everything proceeded in an orderly fashion, in perfect textbook style. CPR, intubation, IV, drugs—we did it all right. Our Medical Director would have been proud. But despite our valiant efforts the little boy died, and I went home that night wondering why…

"Why?" I prayed. "God, why would you allow this to happen?"

My answer never came.

I used to think I knew it all. Not anymore. I'm not even half as smart as I once thought. All I can honestly tell you with certainty is this: There is a God and He's not me, Jesus Christ died for my sins and I'm going to heaven, and my family loves me. And that includes my dog. Other than that, I just don't know. But the good news is God does know. He made the earth and the moon, the sun and the stars. He even made the fabulous Milky Way Galaxy. He created everything there is. That's what I know, and that's all that matters to me.

## PRAYER

Heavenly Father, you created The Milky Way. You created me. You created everything. And that's all I'll ever need to know to trust You with all of my heart.

## APPLICATION

Have you ever stopped to consider the immensity of the universe, or the microscopic worlds teeming within a drop of water? Creation occurred. Nothing is here by mere chance. I once heard someone say, "I don't have enough faith to believe this all just happened." I agree with that statement. Read Genesis 1:1...what does the first verse of the Bible say?

Read the verse again. When did it happen?

Turn in your Bible to Job 36:26. What does this verse say about God?

Go to Job 37:5. What does this passage say about man's understanding of things?

# Answering the Call

Please take a few moments now to read Job 38:1 to 42:3. How does this passage make you feel about God's omnipotence? His understanding?

God created all that there is. He created time. He created you. How should this knowledge affect the way you think about God? The way you respond to His voice?

## BUILDING BLOCKS OF FAITH
If God created the heavens and the earth, He knows all there is to know about you.

# Answering the Call

## JOURNAL

_____

_____

_____

_____

_____

_____

_____

_____

_____

_____

_____

_____

_____

_____

_____

_____

_____

_____

# Welcome Home

Therefore, my brothers, be all the more eager to
make your calling and election sure. For if you do
these things, you will never fall, and you will receive
a rich welcome into the eternal kingdom of our
Lord and Savior Jesus Christ.
2 Peter 1:10-11

It was powerful!

Bagpipes played as the horse drawn caisson rolled past an
army of gray-clad Troopers. Upon its carriage deck lay a
flag covered casket that held the body of an old friend of
mine. A true warrior. A brother in Christ—Trooper 352:
Andrew James Stocks, N.C. Highway Patrol.

We called him A. J.

The Caisson moved quietly to the clicking hooves of six
magnificent black creatures, well groomed horses in regal
parade dress, one without rider to signify loss. The horses
stopped. Six Troopers stepped forward and removed the
casket. They marched quietly into the building and set it
in a place of prominence in the front of the church.

# Answering the Call

The service was awe inspiring, a beautiful memorial to the life of a true first responder—A.J.: U.S. Marine-Crash Firefighter, N.C. Paramedic, N.C. Paramedic Instructor, U.S. Army Ordinance Soldier, and lastly, N.C. State Trooper. Yes, A.J. dedicated his entire career to the service of others. He risked his life so that others might live and, in the end, gave his life selflessly in the line of duty. He was and still is a true hero.

I felt myself jump at the offering of the twenty-one gun salute. Tears filled my eyes as I heard the bagpipes play and the peaceful closing hymns. But I felt my life change at the offering of the radio report that ended the service. A strong male voice came over the air. I felt confused. It surprised me.

"Raleigh, Troop C—"

Silence fell over the room. At first I thought it was a mistake, someone's radio, a Trooper's handheld crackling to life. But then it came again, crisp and clear, a strong voice from somewhere overhead.

"Troop C—"

Dead silence this time. It wasn't a radio; it was a real dispatch going over the air for N.C. Troopers everywhere to hear.

"Troop C...Attention! Trooper 3-5-2 is 10-42."

10-42...*Ending tour of duty.*

# Answering the Call

A. J.'s work on earth was complete, and with that God moved him to his new home in heaven. I know he's there because I asked him one day, "How can you be sure?" He answered, "Because, Pat, I know Jesus Christ died for my sins."

So A. J. has a new home now, and oh what a mansion! Can you imagine it? Built by God's own hands? And it must be marvelous too, for Jesus said, "In my Father's house are many rooms. I am going there to prepare a place for you. I will come back and take you to be with me."

And He did. Jesus came and took my friend home. So wait there for me, brother. Someday Jesus will come to get me too.

## PRAYER

"Thank you for my dear friend, A.J. Now give him a rich welcome, Father, into the eternal kingdom of our Lord and Savior Jesus Christ. May his time in Heaven be as meaningful and passionate as his life was here on earth."

# Answering the Call

## APPLICATION

A.J. understood that Christ died for his sins. He repented and received the gift of eternal life, and in doing so secured for himself a room in God's Heavenly home. You have the same opportunity. Read Acts 2:38-39… what does the scripture say you must do to be saved?

To whom was the promise offered?

In Luke 23:32-43 we see a profound example of Christ's free gift being offered to a guilty man. According to this passage, what must one do in order to follow Christ home, to enter the Kingdom of Heaven?

Now read John 14:2-3. According to this passage, where is Jesus now?

Read Acts 1:9-11. What encouragement did the two angels give Christ's disciples regarding His miraculous departure into Heaven?

# Answering the Call

God created Heaven; it's His; He owns it all. And no one can go to the Father except through His Son, Jesus Christ. Jesus will come back for his children. Will you being going home with him? Will you receive a rich welcome into God's eternal kingdom, or will you spend eternity wondering where you went wrong?

## BUILDING BLOCKS OF FAITH

He who testifies to these things says, "Yes, I am coming soon." Amen. Come, Lord Jesus—Revelation 22:20

## JOURNAL

_____

_____

_____

_____

_____

_____

_____

_____

_____

_____

_____

_____

_____

_____

_____

_____

# Before It's Too Late!

Therefore, get rid of all moral filth and the evil that is so prevalent and humbly accept the word plant- ed in you, which can save you.
James 1:21

"Medic-7, hemorrhage! A 38 year-old female with a severe laceration. Caller reports *heavy bleeding!* Respond Code-3."

My partner and I didn't need to hear the dispatch twice. We jumped into our truck and drove out of the bay. I pushed some buttons and the ambulance lit up like a Christmas tree, lights flashing, siren wailing—Code-3. Bloody images consumed my thoughts as we raced to the call, and as we walked onto the scene those images came to life—a raucous crowd filled a room decorated with bloody wallpaper and jagged pieces of clear broken glass. My patient stood in the center of the room with a blood soaked towel wrapped around her wrist. Crimson drops fell from her fingertips and splattered onto the floor.

I reached for her arm to remove the towel.

"No," someone shouted. "Don't take it off!"

# Answering the Call

"Relax," I said. "I need to see the wound." But as I removed the last of the towel I realized I had made a mistake. A bright red stream spurted from the severed artery, shot across the room, and sprayed the far wall with crimson-colored paint. "Quick," I shouted to my partner. "Hand me a dressing!"

Like my patient, our nation is hemorrhaging. Losing the core values that once made us great. As a people we have become saturated with moral filth. Where are we headed? Will we survive or will God turn His back and leave us to fend for ourselves?

My partner handed me a trauma dressing and a bandage roll, and within seconds I had the wrist tightly wrapped. But the bleeding was far from controlled. Blood continued to drip from her fingertips. Her skin continued to pale.

"Let's go," I said to my partner. "This bleeding must be stopped...before it's too late!"

A moment later we had her in the back of our ambulance with the lights flashing and the siren wailing again—Code-3. I tied the tail of the bandage to the overhead railing hoping that elevating her arm would lessen the flow of blood, but it didn't. I tried using a pressure point, pressing my fingers against the artery above the wound, but the blood still flowed. I had one more option. I wrapped a tourniquet around her arm and tightened it. Finally the bleeding stopped.

# Answering the Call

Is there any dirt in your life? A dark secret or hidden sin? If so your spiritual life is hemorrhaging, keeping you from a closer walk with the Lord.

After starting a large bore IV and administering a fluid bolus, I called the ER to notify them of our arrival. The doctors were waiting for us when we arrived, gloved and gowned in surgical scrubs, ready for business.

"Be careful," I said as an eager resident stepped forward. "This thing will shoot across the room if you take the bandages off."

"Relax," he said with a chuckle. "I got it."

I shrugged and watched him remove the tourniquet. The blood soaked dressings began to drip. He began removing the bandage. I left the room. I couldn't watch.

I returned a few moments later to find an empty room. But the gurney, the floors, the walls—they were covered with blood.

It's time you applied some direct pressure. Get rid of the moral filth in your life. Confess your sins to God. Because once hemorrhage starts it's mighty hard to stop. Humble yourself and turn your face to God…before it's too late.

## PRAYER

"Heavenly Father, I have sinned against You. Plug my wounds. Stop my spiritual hemorrhage. Help me to live a life that is pleasing and honorable to you."

# APPLICATION

How do you think we're doing? As a people? As a nation? Can you list several problems common in our society that are indicative of spiritual hemorrhage?

How about your life? Are you spiritually healthy? What areas of your life could use some hemorrhage control?

What do you believe is to come of our nation if we fail to turn from the path we are now following? What will become of you?

Read 2 Chronicles 7:14. What three things does God say we must do if He is to forgive our sins and heal our land?

What steps will you now take to live a life more pleasing and honorable to God?

# BUILDING BLOCKS OF FAITH

Uncontrolled hemorrhage kills the body. Uncontrolled sin destroys the soul. Learn to master sin, otherwise it will master you.

## JOURNAL

---

---

---

---

---

---

---

---

---

---

---

---

---

# *More Inspirational Books From*
# ❧ **Christian Devotions Books** ❧
### www.christiandevotionsbooks.com

## *Answering the Call -*
### *Inspirational Devotionals from a Tested Paramedic*
### *by Pat Patterson*                                    *Price: $9.95*

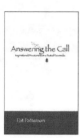

Jesus said, "Greater love has no one than this, that he lay down his life for his friends." The First Responders in your community do just that. They sacrifice comfort and safety to protect the lives of others, always waiting, and always wondering when they will find themselves answering the next call. This book was written for them, but it applies to anyone who searches for courage and hope, struggles with a difficult relationship, or suffers through pain or loss. Are you seeking a closer walk with God? Wondering what comes next? Answering the Call can help you find your way. It reveals the simple truth that Jesus Christ is Lord, and that to follow him is to find true meaning in life. Christ... the First Responder, is calling you now.

*Will you be answering the call? "The promise is for you and your children and for all who are far off -for all whom the Lord our God will call." - Acts 2:39.*

Learn more about this book at: www.answeringthecall.us

## *Faith & FINANCES:*
### *In God We Trust, A Journey to Financial Dependence*
### *by Christian Devotions contributors*          *Price: $9.95*

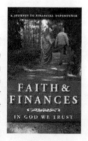

Jesus spoke about money and material possessions more than he talked about heaven, hell, or prayer. He noted the relationship between a man's heart and his wallet, warning, "Where your treasure is, there your heart will be." This contemporary retelling of the Rich Young Ruler brings a fresh look at the relationship between a person's faith and their finances. Within the pages of Faith & FINANCES: In God We Trust you'll find spiritual insight and practical advice from Christy award-winning writer Ann Tatlock, plus best-selling authors, Loree Lough, Yvonne Lehman, Virginia Smith, Irene Brand, DiAnn Mills, Miralee Ferrell, Shelby Rawson and many more.

Great faith calls us to trust God, not our wealth. Read how others have cast off the golden handcuffs and learned to live the abundant life Jesus promised in this contemporary retelling of the Rich Young Ruler. Faith & FINANCES: In God We Trust, A Journey to Financial Dependence - turning the hearts of a nation back toward God one paycheck at a time.

Learn more about this book at: www.faithandfinances.us

## *Spirit & HEART: A Devotional Journey*
### *by Christian Devotions contributors*    Price: $9.95

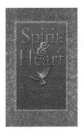

What is a devotional journey? It is the Bible. Today we enjoy the benefit of the prayers, wisdom, praise and sorrow of people who, during their lifetime, chose to remember the times God worked in their lives. That is devotion to God and dedication to recording "His Story." The daily devotions included in this book are heartfelt stories, lessons, and advice from others who have traveled the devotional journey. This book is a primer, a tool to get you started on the path toward spending your best moments with the Father. Christ says, where your heart is there your treasure will be. Treasure His words and whispers as you walk in the footsteps of award-winning authors Ann Tatlock, Loree Lough, Yvonne Lehman, Virginia Smith, Irene Brand, Shelby Rawson, Eddie Jones, Cindy Sproles, Ariel Allison-plus many more.

Learn more about this book at: www.devotionsbook.com

## *Emerson The Magnificent!*
### *by Dwight Ritter*                Price: $12.99

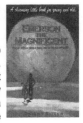

"A charming little book for young and old."

How an old bike takes a young man for the ride of his life.

"What a delight... though I thought it unlikely that a bicycle could do much to unravel some complicated issues, my skepticism was outvoted. It really doesn't matter how old you are, Emerson talks to you. Dwight Ritter's illustrations made me smile as much as his story warmed my heart. Emerson's message challenged my thinking, then threw me a lifeline, reeled me in and rescued me. Get it! Read it! Give it to everyone you know! " - by Pat Lindquist.

Learn more about this book at: www.emersonthemagnificent.com

**More Inspirational Books Available From**
**Christian Devotions Ministry's Book Division**
**www.christiandevotionsbooks.com**

Made in the USA
Lexington, KY
04 May 2015